UNMASKING
SUPER
FOODS

UNMASKING
SUPER
FOODS

THE TRUTH AND HYPE ABOUT
AÇAÍ, QUINOA, CHIA, BLUEBERRIES, AND MORE

JENNIFER SYGO, MSc, RD

Collins

Published by Collins, an imprint of HarperCollins Publishers Ltd.

Unless otherwise noted, all nutrition information is derived from the USDA National
Nutrient Database, with percentages of daily values obtained from nutritiondata.com.
Although serving sizes used in this book tend to be 1 cup for fruits, vegetables, and cooked
grains, it should be noted that these serving sizes represent, in many cases, two servings
according to *Canada's Food Guide* (for example, a serving of fruit or vegetables is 1/2 cup,
except for leafy or salad greens, in which case a serving is 1 cup; likewise, a serving of cooked
grain, such as quinoa, is usually 1/2 cup).

HarperCollins books may be purchased for educational, business, or sales promotional use
through our Special Markets Department.

HarperCollins Publishers Ltd
2 Bloor Street East, 20th Floor
Toronto, Ontario, Canada
M4W 1A8

www.harpercollins.ca

Library and Archives Canada Cataloguing in Publication information is available upon
request.
ISBN 978-1-44341-978-9

Printed and bound in the United States
RRD 9 8 7 6 5 4 3

For Dave, Ben, and Ryan, for making every day better.
And to my mom and dad: Thanks for reminding me that
the long-distance runner wins in the end.

CONTENTS

Introduction   1

1 Overhyped, Overpriced, or Just Plain Bogus: 5
   How Industry Corrupted the Superfood Movement

2 Quinoa, I Thought I Knew Ya: 41
   Superfoods with Question Marks

3 Smear Campaign: 78
   Superfoods with an Unfairly Bad Rap

4 Classics!   124
   Superfoods That Still Rule

5 Send Me a Hero: 207
   Overlooked and Underappreciated Superfoods

Conclusion   239
Acknowledgements   241
Notes   243
Index   277

INTRODUCTION

Flaxseed is so 2006. If I had written this book just a few years ago, I would probably have written about flaxseed. But in 2014, flaxseed is so obvious it's almost, like, *yawn.* I can actually picture hipsters of the future dusting off a package of flaxseed and setting off a frenzy of flaxseed collecting. Like drinking Fanta, eating flaxseed would be steeped in yesteryear irony, a time before we spent our free moments debating about whether or not our sprouted gluten-free grains are Paleo, or if there is such thing as an ethical carnivore.

Ironically, considering this book's title, I actually struggle with the term *superfood*. Maybe it's the Marxist in me, but I'm concerned that it unfairly elevates certain foods above others, leaving us to feel that if our favourite veggie isn't on the list, then it must not have much value. Poor celery! I just don't think that attitude is fair or wise. The fact is, for all of our perceived cleverness, we simply don't know that much about our food, and we certainly don't know enough to say exactly what makes a true "superfood." Even the ones that seem the most nutritious have precious little research to tell us whether those extra nutrients translate into anything particularly meaningful; and sometimes, foods that look a little average on paper—strawberries, I'm looking at you—seem to have pretty clear health benefits. I also balk at making eating and nutrition some kind of competitive sport, where your kale-based smoothie somehow makes you better than me, because I'm "only" munching on carrot sticks. If we need to feel sorry for someone because they don't own a $700 blender to emulsify a week's worth of groceries, I think we've probably taken a good thing too far. And I'm afraid the superfood movement might well be feeding into that.

Thankfully, we might finally be starting to appreciate the elegant complexity of food in its undoctored form. Whole foods have literally hundreds, even thousands, of active compounds, including phenolics, flavonoids, pigments, antioxidants, fatty acids, protein, vitamins, minerals, fibre, and resistant starches—the list goes on and on—and it is the interaction of these nutrients that makes whole foods so special. But to pretend that we know exactly what makes one food "super" and another, well, "average" is downright silly. There is too much left to learn, and, frankly, the whole challenge of understanding food is so massively complex that I think we're unlikely to ever get to the bottom of it (but hats off to all the good researchers who are devoting their life's work to trying).

As a result, it is not my aim in this book to create a ranking system of superfoods, although there have been times when I've been tempted (it's hard not to start mentally awarding gold medals when you see just how magnificent the nutrition profile of kale is). I'm also not going to pretend this book is in any way a complete picture of all the foods that could somehow be labelled "super"; basically, you could take any list of whole foods that walk, fly, swim, or grow and make the case that somehow, in some way, they qualify. In fact, some classic superfoods, such as salmon, olive oil, and yogurt, didn't even make it into this book, simply because they have been covered so well elsewhere, and if I didn't stop somewhere, this book could have gone on forever.

What I do want to do, however, is turn a critical eye to all the hype that surrounds so many so-called superfoods. Is there good reason for us to jump off the deep end every time we come across an obscure Himalayan berry? Will paying $40 for a litre of juice really make us live longer? And what about common foods that are both affordable and accessible? Are they any less worthy of our affection? These are important questions in the emerging multi-billion-dollar health food industry.

This book is divided into five sections. The first looks at superfoods that have fallen on the wrong side of the regulators or even the law; it should serve as a cautionary tale about the consequences of us all getting a little drunk on the latest food craze. The second part of the book is devoted to foods that have earned a good chunk of hype, yet are so poorly understood that we should approach them with a dose of caution until we know more. The third section is all about the dirty pleasures of the superfood world—superfoods that have been cast aside in the press or the medical literature and yet might have more to offer than their reputation suggests. The fourth section is all about some of the classic superfoods, but with careful consideration of what we really know about them and where our false assumptions lie, while the last part of *Unmasking Superfoods* looks at certain foods that might not have the exotic appeal of goji berries but deserve more attention than they get.

1

OVERHYPED, OVERPRICED, OR JUST PLAIN BOGUS

HOW INDUSTRY CORRUPTED THE SUPERFOOD MOVEMENT

The superfood movement is ripe for fraud. With a growing consumer population keen on fixing all that ails us through food, the goal is simple: Find the most nutrient-rich foods you can, and eat as much of them as possible. Now, this is all well and good when we're talking about apples and broccoli—foods that are readily accessible, grown locally, and generally affordable. The picture muddies, however, when we fall in love with rare and mysterious foods (most often a berry) from a land far away, with tales of healing powers and the ability to provide boundless vitality. *Amazing*, we think. *One shot of this per day and I'll finally get a six-pack, clean out the garage, and maybe even run across the Sahara.* Brilliant! And really, who couldn't use more energy? Forty bucks doesn't seem unreasonable to cure arthritis, eczema, insomnia, low sex drive, and wrinkles. How could it? You're worth it! And while you're at it, since it'll help prevent cancer, heart attacks, and Alzheimer's disease, maybe you should take two.

The nutrients, the antioxidants, and the health claims associated with so many superfoods often sound too good to be true, and if the testimonials are convincing enough, we might just find ourselves handing over our credit cards for a month's supply of a drink, powder, or potion. And we might just feel better when we take it—for a while.

If you're a savvy food marketer or business person who has an interest in the massive health and wellness market, you'd probably like to get one of these so-called superfoods into consumer hands, and ideally, make a few bucks in the process. Of course, geography poses a problem: It's not so easy to get a Himalayan berry onto grocery store shelves halfway around the world. So, if you can't sell it fresh, then what? You turn it into a powder, pill, or juice, but that increases production costs—so you'd better have a good marketing strategy to convince the public it's worth spending their hard-earned cash on. This is the reality in a competitive health food industry: You have to do something to get your product noticed. The best way to do that? Tell the world your food cures just about everything, or get it on TV (*The Dr. Oz Show* is a great place to start).

This chapter is all about foods that found themselves on both sides of the superfood hype machine: built up by promises of nutritional greatness and then brought back to earth by investigative journalism, FDA warning letters, and in some cases, lawsuits. For better or for worse, these foods, in their original form, might actually be quite good for you; unfortunately, that feel-good quality tends to get lost when the cease and desist orders are issued and when consumers are duped by misleading or fraudulent claims.

AÇAÍ

If there is a food that serves as the blueprint for superfood hype, it might just be açaí. Unheard of in North America until just a few years ago, açaí (pronounced ah-SIGH-ee) made its way onto the North American radar in 2008 when famed physician Dr. Mehmet Oz appeared on *The Oprah Winfrey Show* and touted açaí among his "anti-aging checklist."[1] With ringing endorsements from the likes of dermatologist Dr. Nicholas Perricone (a frequent guest of Oprah's who ranked açaí as his number one superfood[2]), açaí rocketed from obscurity to ubiquity in an Internet heartbeat.

AÇAÍ: THE STORY

Açaí berries are the fruit of the Brazilian palm *Euterpe oleracea* Martius. With a long history of use for traditional healing, much of açaí's popularity, which reportedly reached US$104 million in 2008,[3] centred around its purported weight-loss benefits, though other claims have been made relating to heart health, muscle and joint pain relief, and cancer prevention. Although açaí naturally exists as a small purple berry, it is most commonly consumed in North America as a component of blended fruit juices. When it first emerged on the market, much of the açaí available was distributed through a company known as MonaVie, which sold açaí juice as part of a mixed blend of juices on a multi-level marketing platform—at a cost of $40 per bottle. Yes, you read that right: For the same amount of money as would be needed to feed a family of four fresh produce for a week, you could get a bottle of fruit juice. Since then, açaí has found its way into numerous popular products, including smoothies, fruit juice blends, weight-loss supplements, and Dr. Perricone's recommended vehicle, as açaí powder.

HOW MUCH FOR A BOTTLE OF AÇAÍ?

How much fresh produce could you get for the price of a bottle of mixed açaí juice? Here's a breakdown, based on a local grocery store's prices.

AÇAÍ VERSUS YOUR LOCAL GROCERY STORE

ITEM	UNIT COST	AMOUNT	SUBTOTAL
Bananas	$0.69/lb	2 lb	$1.38
Apples	$1.49/lb	3 lb	$4.47
Carrots	$1.99/bunch (5–6 carrots)	1 bunch	$1.99
Celery	$1.99/bunch	1 bunch	$1.99
Romaine lettuce	$1.49/head	1 head	$1.49
Blueberries	$3.99/pint	1 pint	$3.99
Tomatoes	$1.29/lb	2 large (1/2 lb)	$0.65
Mushrooms	$2.99/lb	1/4 lb	$0.75
Kale	$1.99/bunch	1 bunch	$1.99
Broccoli	$2.49/bunch	1 bunch	$2.49
Green beans	$2.49/lb	1 lb	$2.49
Onions	$1.29/lb	3 medium (3/4 lb)	$0.97
Cucumber	$1.29/item	1 cucumber	$1.29
Pears	$1.49/lb	3 pears (1.5 lb)	$2.24
Grapes	$2.29/lb	2 lb	$4.58
Potatoes	$1.29/lb	2 lb	$2.58
Sweet potatoes	$1.29/lb	2 lb	$2.58
Oranges	$1.29/lb	2 lb	$2.58
			TOTAL $40.50

So, for the same cost as a single bottle of blended açaí juice, you could get not only enough produce to feed a family of four for a week but also substantially more nutrition, including more vitamins A and C, potassium, folate, and fibre, than you would in a whole bottle of the juice.

AÇAÍ: THE NUTRITION

For all the hype surrounding açaí's potential to influence our health or our weight, one would expect it to have a fairly attractive nutrition profile. In reality, however, we know very little about açaí, other than what we can glean from a handful of journal articles and industry-sponsored websites, much of which relates to blended juices that are not pure açaí. According to Sambazon, a supplier of açaí juice (Sambazon is short for Saving and Managing the Brazilian Amazon), an 8 ounce serving of Açaí: The Original juice (which is made from açaí berry juice, agave sweetener, and lime juice—more on agave later) provides 140 calories' worth of energy, along with 3 grams of fat and 1 gram of protein.[4] Of its 28 grams of carbohydrate, a single gram is from fibre (by comparison, we should be aiming for 25 to 38 grams per day), and 24 grams is sugar. Aside from the slightly higher fat content, these numbers are about the same as you would find in any berry or grape juice—in other words, unremarkable.

As for vitamins and minerals, Sambazon's juice provides 6% of our daily vitamin A needs (by comparison, a carrot will give you a whole day's worth of vitamin A), 6% of your calcium, and 4% of your daily iron needs. It also provides 75 mg of potassium, which is about the same as you'd get in a bite of banana. In other words, if there is something special about açaí, it's not its vitamins and minerals.

Enter the antioxidants. According to popular theory, the health benefits of fruits, vegetables, and other plant foods are derived less from vitamins and minerals and more from compounds known as polyphenols and flavonoids, which are thought to act as antioxidants in our bodies. As the story goes, age, pollution, and exposure to UV light, among other things, are associated with a process known as oxidation in our bodies. This oxidation leads to the production of free radicals, harmful compounds that are thought to damage our cells over time, eventually contributing to everything from wrinkles to heart disease to cancer.

Following that logic, anything that can slow down, stop, or reverse oxidation and the production of free radicals in our bodies would be considered a possible disease fighter. Makers of açaí products often claim that açaí is one of the most antioxidant-rich foods around, and in particular it is a source of the same bluish-purple antioxidants found in blueberries, known as anthocyanins.[5,6] That sounds promising—but, as you'll see, the reality is somewhat less sensational.

Antioxidant capacity can be measured a few different ways, perhaps most commonly using the oxygen radical absorbance capacity, or ORAC, score. Basically, ORAC allows us to directly compare the antioxidant activity of one food against another, with the assumption that the food with the higher ORAC would be the healthiest, most disease-fighting food. In reality, we have precious little evidence that a high ORAC score translates into any *real* (versus theoretical) health benefit. The evidence is so shaky that the United States Department of Agriculture (USDA) removed the ORAC Database for Selected Foods from its Nutrient Data Laboratory website "due to mounting evidence that the values indicating antioxidant capacity have no relevance to the effects of specific bioactive compounds, including polyphenols, on human health."[7] Oops. Taking it a step further, the U.S. Food and Drug Administration (FDA) also cautioned that "ORAC values are routinely misused by food and dietary supplement manufacturing companies to promote their products and by consumers to guide their food and dietary supplement choices." Double oops. So, even if açaí is the gold standard for antioxidants, the truth is we really have no good evidence that it will make us any healthier in the long run.

But if we pretend, just for a moment, that ORAC is a serious tool for assessing nutritional value in a food, then it is probably worth mentioning that a 2008 study, published in the *Journal of Agriculture and Food Chemistry*, found that when it comes to both antioxidant content and function, açaí juice actually falls unremarkably in the middle of the pack, ahead of cranberry, orange, and apple juice but behind pomegranate juice, red wine, and concord grape juice.[8]

So much for the hype.

AÇAÍ: THE SCIENCE

For all the attention afforded to açaí, it might surprise you to know there is almost no research on this so-called superfood. In one of the few human studies to date, published in the *Journal of Agriculture and Food Chemistry* in 2008, researchers asked 12 healthy subjects to drink MonaVie and then measured the antioxidant status in their bloodstreams for the next two hours.[9] Although the subjects did see some improvements in their antioxidant status in the short term after drinking MonaVie, as you can probably already guess, there's nothing to connect that to any real effect on our overall health.

Aside from this single trial, a small number of pilot studies have investigated the impact of various açaí products on subjects' health, though many have been industry sponsored and published in smaller, lower-quality journals. Importantly, pilot studies are not blinded, meaning the researchers, and often the subjects, are aware of what they are taking during the trial, which means the results are far more likely to be skewed in favour of the product or supplement than if those involved in the study were unaware of who was taking what. In other words, we can't take much from the results of pilot studies on açaí, or any other food or supplement; their role is to serve as a jumping-off point for more research.

And what of the claims of açaí's role in weight loss? At this time, no study has been published to suggest that consuming açaí in any form will help you lose weight or shed body fat.

AÇAÍ SIDE EFFECTS?

There are few downsides to eating berries or enjoying moderate portions of their juices, but a case of rhabdomyolysis, a serious condition characterized by muscle breakdown and possible kidney damage, has been reported in a young male taking an açaí-based weight-loss supplement for two weeks.[10] Although researchers traced the subject's condition back to his use of the supplement, ironically, when the drink was tested, the researchers found it contained no significant levels of açaí juice.

THE BOTTOM LINE

A recent review published in the journal *Phytochemical Letters* stated it well: "[açaí] is a poster child of the power of the Internet to promote products for which only limited phytochemical and pharmacological information is available."[11] Like any berry, the fruit of the açaí palm tree does have some nutritional value, but so far, we have no good evidence to say it's different from virtually most other commonly available fruits and vegetables. Any other statements as to its possible role in weight control, heart disease prevention, muscle and joint health, or cancer prevention are, at this time, unsubstantiated. What we do know is that the hype around açaí has meant big business for some and a lot of money out of the pockets of others.

MULTI-LEVEL MARKETING

In 2007, the FDA issued a warning to the producers of MonaVie, a distributor of açaí juice, that the claims made on their website, acaiberry.com, relating to several products in the MonaVie line, were in violation of the Federal Food, Drug, and Cosmetic Act and that the MonaVie products "are not generally recognized as safe and effective for the above referenced conditions," including cholesterol management and relief of joint and muscle pain and inflammation.[12] Even without the warning, MonaVie had drawn criticism for its business model based on multi-level marketing (MLM), which some critics argue resembles a pyramid scheme.[13] In 2009, Harpo, Inc., the producers of *The Oprah Winfrey Show* and *The Dr. Oz Show*, filed a complaint against 40 Internet marketers of dietary supplements, including açaí, for using both Winfrey's and Oz's images without consent to promote their products.[14] The case was eventually settled out of court. Earlier that same year, the Centre for Science in the Public Interest (CSPI), a food and nutrition watchdog, published a warning to readers about Internet scams related to açaí.[15] According to the CSPI, which published the warning in its periodical, *Nutrition Action Healthletter*, when customers purchased açaí products online, even for a free trial, they were often charged for products they had not ordered, and cancelling was nearly impossible.

GOJI

Like açaí, goji berries hit the motherlode when they were featured on *The Oprah Winfrey Show*. On a 2007 episode featuring Chicago Bulls basketball star Ben Gordon seeking nutrition advice to help him manage his at times thrice-daily workouts, Dr. Oz advised Gordon he would benefit from reducing oxidation building up in his muscles by consuming more antioxidant-rich foods. And, according to Oz, the Himalayan goji berry is "the most potent antioxidant fruit that we know."[16] And so, a star was born.

GOJI: THE STORY

Goji berries, also known as wolfberries, are the fruit of the *Lycium barbarum* or *L. chinense* plant. Native to southeastern Europe and Asia, goji berries are largely imported from China and the Himalayas, where they have been used in traditional Chinese medicine. They are thought to help improve diabetes management and support a healthy immune system while also providing less tangible benefits, such as increased energy and vitality.

Although goji berries can be eaten raw, they are typically available in North America in dried or powdered form. With an appearance like a reddish-orange raisin and a slightly bittersweet taste, dried goji berries are often used in trail mixes and in cold or hot cereal. You can also find goji teas, and you can soak the dried fruit in hot water to make a plump berry.

Like açaí juice, goji berries and juices aren't gentle on the pocketbook: A 500-gram bag can cost up to $40 at health food stores. Navitas Naturals, purveyor of prepackaged superfoods, sells goji in 4-ounce ($5.99), 8-ounce ($10.99), and 16-ounce ($20.99) bags. The good news? You get free shipping for orders over $70.[17]

GOJI TROUBLE

Goji juice, in various forms, is available from numerous websites, often as part of multi-level marketing platforms. Some distributors of goji berries have also landed themselves in trouble with the FDA for making claims that are consistent with drugs.[18] In 2009, a lawsuit was brought against FreeLife International on the grounds of "misrepresentation and deception in the marketing and sale" of some goji products.[19] Among FreeLife's products? Himalayan Goji Juice, GoChi Juice, and a goji-based weight-loss supplement known as TAIslim.

GOJI: THE NUTRITION

Tracking down reliable nutrition information for goji berries is not an easy task since they are not found in the Canadian Nutrient File[20] or USDA National Nutrient Database.[21] The only nutrition information available is from suppliers, and with that comes a substantial amount of variability from site to site. According to Navitas Naturals, goji berries provide "18 amino acids, free-radical fighting antioxidants, carotenoids, vitamins A, C, and E, and more than 20 other trace minerals and vitamins including zinc, iron, phosphorus, and riboflavin (B_2)."[22] The company also claims that "Ounce-for-ounce, goji berries contain more vitamin C than oranges, more beta-carotene than carrots, and more iron than soybeans and spinach."

That sounds great. The only problem is that we have to take the manufacturer's word for it; there's no way to verify how much of this information is true. The Nutrition Facts table for Navitas Naturals' goji berries purports that 1 ounce (28 grams) of dried berries provides 100 calories' worth of energy, along with 0 grams of fat (which sort of flies in the face of their claims that goji is a source of essential fatty acids, unless they exist at minuscule, and therefore virtually irrelevant, levels). You'll also obtain 21 grams of carbohydrate, a respectable 3 grams of fibre, and 4 grams of protein, or about the same as you'll get from 1/4 cup of beans or chickpeas, which by comparison will cost you about a dime.

If goji has any real bragging rights, it's probably related to its vitamin A content (140% of your daily needs per serving of dried berries), which is in the same realm as various other orange and red fruits and vegetables. All that vitamin A comes at a cost, however: An ounce of goji berries contains 75 more calories than a medium carrot and yet provides only two-thirds as much vitamin A. And while an ounce of goji might provide more vitamin C, gram for gram, than an orange, if we compare realistic portions, you'd have to eat 5 ounces of goji berries to get the 106% of your daily vitamin C that an orange provides, packing in a near Big Mac–worthy 500 calories (versus 60 to 80 for an orange) and costing your pocketbook about $7.50.

GOJI: THE SCIENCE

To date, all the double-blind, placebo-controlled trials—the gold standard of clinical research—on the possible benefits of goji berries or juice have been conducted by two companies that, as luck would have it, manufacture goji-related products. The first group of studies has been published by none other than the makers of GoChi, the same group who faced a lawsuit for "misrepresentation and deception in the marketing and sale" of their goji products. They have published four trials on their juice that, perhaps not surprisingly, have all had favourable results. In the first, published in the *Journal of Alternative and Complementary Medicine* in 2008, subjects who drank 1/2 cup of GoChi per day for two weeks reported "increased ratings for energy level, athletic performance, quality of sleep, ease of awakening, ability to focus on activities, mental acuity, calmness, and feelings of health" versus placebo.[23] Although this sounds like a rather ringing endorsement for goji, these are entirely subjective measures. The absence of any objective measures, such as blood pressure or cholesterol, renders these results virtually irrelevant.

In a follow-up study, a group of 50 Chinese adults given 1/2 cup of goji juice every day for a month had higher levels of antioxidant markers (known as superoxide dismutase, or SOD, and glutathione peroxidase, or GSH-Px) than those on a placebo.[24] They also had less damage (peroxidation) to some of their circulating fats (known as lipids). Unfortunately, that's all we know: We have no idea how these antioxidant levels compare with other berries or fruits, or if they correspond to any long-term (or even short-term) health benefit. The bottom line? Although the makers of GoChi would like you to believe otherwise, they haven't proven—or even convincingly suggested—that goji does much of anything to make us healthier.

The second group studying goji, based out of Switzerland, make a proprietary milk-based formulation of goji, known as Lacto-Wolfberry, and have used it in studies on macular degeneration, a degenerative eye disease that can lead to loss of vision, especially in the elderly. After three months, subjects taking the drink had higher circulating levels of zeaxanthin, a compound also found in egg yolks and thought to play a role in eye health and possibly in the prevention of macular degeneration. However, the researchers were unable to say whether the supplement actually prevented or slowed the progression of the disease.[25]

And what about goji for weight loss? To date, the only study conducted on humans has been published by—you guessed it—the makers of GoChi. In this study on 29 otherwise healthy overweight adults, those given 4 ounces (120 ml) of GoChi per day saw their waistlines shrink by about 5 cm (2 inches) after two weeks versus those taking a placebo (dummy drink).[26] How is that possible? The researchers found that those taking GoChi burned 10% more calories (known as post-prandial energy expenditure) in the hour after taking 1/2 cup of GoChi. Although these results suggest that goji juice *could* contribute to weight loss by helping us burn extra energy at rest, they need to be validated by other longer-term studies, conducted by independent research groups, to determine exactly how meaningful they are.

GOJI SIDE EFFECTS?

As a point of caution, Health Canada has added goji to the list of natural health and food products that can interfere with the drug warfarin, a commonly prescribed blood thinner.[27] There have also been reported cases of allergic reactions to goji, one of which was anaphylactic.[28] The reaction seems to be triggered by a protein shared by both goji and tomatoes, which are part of the same family of plants. A single case of sun allergy, also known as photosensitivity, has been reported in a man taking goji berries for five months.[29] Although the allergic and sun reactions to goji are rare, since it is a relatively unstudied fruit, other reactions to goji may not have yet been reported.

THE BOTTOM LINE

You might say that goji berries are a "nice to have" but not a "need to have." Like all berries, they do seem to have some redeeming nutritional value—they are high in vitamin A, for example—but whether or not they have special benefits that make them worth the extra cash is unclear at best. What is certain is that, like açaí, goji is backed by a small body of industry-sponsored research, as well as large-scale Internet hype, and costs a pretty penny to boot.

NONI JUICE

How can a small, utterly unpalatable berry migrate halfway around the world, becoming a semi-household name and igniting a multi-million-dollar industry in the process? Through the power of Internet marketing, of course. Noni, the South Pacific superfood, became a darling in much the same way as goji and açaí (though without the ringing endorsement on *Oprah*): via outrageous testimonials, Internet chatter, and multi-level marketing. There might not be any good evidence to support the claims associated with noni, but that hasn't stopped dozens of noni-containing products from flooding the market.

NONI: THE STORY

The noni plant, also known as *Morinda citrifolia* L., or Indian mulberry, is a plant whose fruit, bark, and leaves are used in traditional healing in French Polynesia, Hawaii, and other parts of the South Pacific to treat a wide range of conditions, including chronic pain, arthritis, diabetes, high blood pressure, asthma, and infection.[30] Noni's transition from traditional medicine to mainstream supplement began when the late Dr. Ralph Heinicke, a researcher for the Dole Pineapple Company and the University of Hawaii, found that pineapple and noni shared an active compound, which his research suggested could have medicinal properties. In 1983, Dr. Heinicke patented this compound, known as xeronine, which he claimed noni possessed in large quantities.

Since then, noni has been sold in North America primarily as a juice or juice blend or as an extract that is taken orally. In general, the doses recommended by marketers of noni products are small—one ounce (30 ml) taken twice daily, which is about all that most people can afford: According to the Morinda Bioactives website, a 1 L glass bottle of Tahitian Noni retails for $38, though the unit price mercifully goes down when you buy in bulk.[31] Pure noni juice is known for its less-than-pleasant taste, which means that much of the noni on the market is made from blended juices, making it difficult to know just how much noni you are getting from your drink.

NAUGHTY NONI

Like açaí and goji juice, many noni products were originally distributed via multi-level marketing, and as with the other players in the multi-level exotic berry market, noni distributors ran into trouble with U.S. regulators, who warned makers of Tahitian Noni (now Morinda Bioactives) that their product claims were not backed by adequate research and crossed the line into the territory of a drug rather than a food.[32] Now readily available from multiple distributors, including popular retail chains, noni-related products had estimated sales of US$250 million by 2005.[33]

NONI: THE NUTRITION

As with other exotic berries on MLM platforms, there is limited information on the nutritional makeup of noni juice. According to Morinda Bioactives, a 30 ml (1 ounce) serving of noni juice provides 10 calories' worth of energy and 3 grams of carbohydrate, of which 2 grams come from sugar. Aside from its basic nutrition profile, a recent analysis of noni juice found that it possesses antioxidant properties, particularly through its vitamin C content, as well as compounds known as phenols and iridoids. It also might have some anti-inflammatory effects.[34] And that's all we know.

NONI: THE SCIENCE

To date, there have been no randomized, double-blind, placebo-controlled trials demonstrating that noni has any impact on long-term human health. Not one. The small number of trials that have been conducted have either been on very specific issues (post-operative nausea and vomiting, or dental irrigation, anyone?) or in lower-quality journals. Aside from randomized controlled trials (RCTs), there is a fairly significant amount of research on animals and cell lines (studies conducted at the cellular level) suggesting that noni could have heart health benefits (in hamsters) and antimicrobial effects (it can wage a hearty battle against fecal matter in test tubes), can upregulate the immune system, and can protect against certain cancers (in mice). Unfortunately, much of this work has been industry funded or poorly controlled—and none has been replicated in humans.

Noni does seem to exert an effect on a compound known as nitric oxide (NO), which has been linked with blood pressure control, erectile health, and performance benefits for athletes. To date, however, only one study has been conducted on the effects of noni in athletic performance, and that was on rats given Tahitian Noni Juice before a swim test.[35] To their credit, the rats given the noni took longer to fatigue than their controls, but there is much more research needed in the area before we have any idea how this translates to humans.

And before you say, "What's the harm?" when it comes to trying noni, remember this: The most common side effect associated with noni juice is liver toxicity, which has been reported in at least a half-dozen cases.[36]

THE BOTTOM LINE

Although non-human research has shown that noni could have some health benefits, the same has been said about dozens, even hundreds, of other foods, supplements, and products over the years. Until we have some data in humans, it is far too early to say what, exactly, noni juice can and should be used for—other than to serve as a very expensive fruit drink.

COCONUT WATER

Looking to wet your whistle with something lighter than coconut milk? Want to hang with all the hot celebrities? Feel like this is the year you'll finally run that ultra-marathon? Consider coconut water. At least that's the public image of this massively popular pseudo–sports drink.

COCONUT WATER: THE STORY

If you popped a straw inside an immature (green) coconut, the liquid you would be sipping would be coconut water, the megadrink that has enjoyed the backing of the likes of Madonna and Rihanna (no word on support from other single-moniker stars Cher and Beyoncé). Although coconut water can be enjoyed straight from a coconut, the image of sipping a large brown-husked fruit on the subway lacks a certain convenience; hence, the introduction of cans and Tetra Paks, which have become vehicles for the drink whose sales are said to have exceeded US$350 million per year.[37] Coconut water can now be found in health food stores, grocery stores, and gas station convenience stores alike. It's everywhere.

COCONUT WATER: THE NUTRITION

A cup of coconut water provides only half the calories of most varieties of pop, at 46 per 8-ounce (237 ml) serving. It also provides 9 grams of carbohydrate, of which 6 grams are sugar and 3 grams are fibre (full marks there: that's an unusually high fibre content for a drink), along with 2 grams of protein. In terms of vitamins, coconut water offers up 10% of your vitamin C (less than the amount in an orange slice), a pinch of B vitamins, and a splash of calcium (58 mg, or 6% of your 1,000 mg daily needs). Coconut water's big claim to fame is its potassium content, providing 17% (600 mg) of your daily value—that's almost as much potassium as a potato or sweet potato and more than a banana.

COCONUT WATER VERSUS SPORTS DRINKS

BEVERAGE TYPE	Gatorade	Powerade	Vita Coco	O.N.E.
Portion size (ml)	355	360	255	330
Calories per serving	80	80	45	60
Carbohydrate (g/serving)	21	21	11	14
Carbohydrate (g/100 ml)*	5.9	5.8	4.3	4.2
Sodium (mg/serving)	160	150	30	65
Sodium (mg/100 ml)†	45	42	12	20
Potassium (mg)	45	35	470	610

Source: Manufacturers' websites

*target = 4–8 g/100 ml
†target = 50–70 mg/100 ml

The affection for coconut water is several-fold: Not only is it a low-calorie beverage, but the combination of moderate sugar and high potassium—an electrolyte, or salt, that is lost in sweat—has made coconut water a postmodern sports drink sensation. In a world where added sugars, artificial colours, and sodium are increasingly frowned upon, coconut water lets athletes feel good about fueling their bodies with something natural.

Coconut water is usually sold in bottles, cans, or Tetra Paks, ranging in volume from 330 to 414 ml, at a cost of about $2.50 per serving. Although the taste of coconut water varies by brand, its flavour is not necessarily a welcome one for the North American palate. As a result, many companies are introducing coconut water blends to the market, which can translate to less coconut water and more added sugar.

COCONUT WATER: THE SCIENCE

So, is there reason to believe that coconut water is the real deal, at least for athletes? In the first known study comparing it with a common sports drink, coconut water proved just as effective for rehydrating treadmill runners after a 90-minute run.[38] One other study suggested it may be better tolerated (meaning it caused less nausea and stomach upset), compared with a sports drink or plain water, when consumed after intense exercise.[39]

Those are both interesting findings, but that doesn't mean coconut water is the ideal sports drink to be consumed *during* sports. Although it's generally accepted that plain water is fine for activities lasting up to around 90 minutes, it is in longer training or competition settings that an athlete may need to start taking in some carbohydrate to keep from "hitting the wall," or "bonking." Technically speaking, bonking happens when athletes run out of quick-burning carbohydrates in their muscles. They feel exhausted, and they have no choice but to slow down. To stave off hitting the wall, athletes are supposed to take in about 30 to 60 grams of carbohydrate per hour, either through food, such as bananas, or liquids, such as sports drinks.[40] If athletes do use a sports drink, the carbohydrate concentration is crucial: ideally, it shoud be somewhere between 4 and 8 grams per 100 ml of fluid (also known as a 4% to 8% carbohydrate drink), which mimics the natural concentration of sugar in the bloodstream.[41] This is where coconut water falls short: It provides just 9 grams of carbohydrate per 250 ml, or 3.6 grams of carbohydrate per 100 ml. In other words, when it comes to pushing back "the wall," coconut water won't cut it for long.

Coconut water also falls short when it comes to sodium. Although sodium might be a nutrient most of us could stand to reduce, for athletes, it can be vital for performance. Why? Because it's lost in sweat, and if an athlete's blood levels of sodium drop too low, they run the risk not only of cramping but also of developing hyponatremia, or low sodium in the bloodstream. Hyponatremia, which may be becoming more common as slower athletes take the hydration message too far and actually overhydrate during endurance events such as marathons, can be just as dangerous as dehydration, and it can even be deadly. To help replenish some of the salt lost in sweat, and therefore to hopefully reduce some of the risk of hyponatremia, it's recommended that athletes take in 300 to 700 mg of sodium for every litre of fluid they drink. As for coconut water? It provides less than half that amount.[42] It shouldn't be surprising, then, that the likes of tennis player John Isner, who is sponsored by Vita Coco, is said to have added salt to his coconut water to get him through the longest match in the history of professional tennis.[43, 44]

COCONUT WATER CONTROVERSY

All this talk of coconut water's nutrition is fine in theory, as long as you're drinking your coconut water straight out of a coconut (as the researchers in the running study did). In a review published in August 2011, however, Consumer Lab found that, among three major U.S. brands of coconut water—Vita Coco (distributed through the Dr Pepper Snapple Group Inc.), O.N.E. Coconut Water (purchased by Pepsi in 2010), and Zico Natural (scooped up by Coke in 2009 for $15 million)—only Zico Natural lived up to its labelling claims, at least in terms of sugar, sodium, potassium, and magnesium.[45] The other two fell short in two or more categories: Vita Coco, which boasts Demi Moore and Madonna as investors, contained only 59% of the sodium and 64% of the magnesium claimed on its labels, while O.N.E. contained a mere 18% of the sodium and 77% of the magnesium, amounts that fall outside the FDA's accepted 20% variation for natural foods. Although less sodium would seem to be a plus, many of the claims related to coconut water centre around its role in improving hydration during and recovery from strenuous activity; in that role, sodium is thought to play an important role in boosting performance.

As a result of Consumer Lab's report, a class-action lawsuit was launched against Vita Coco. In the settlement, Vita Coco agreed to change its packaging and remove comparisons to sports drinks, including statements claiming that Vita Coco contains "15 times the potassium found in leading sports drinks."[46] They also agreed to improve quality control, including more regular testing of their products to ensure accuracy. In the meantime, consumers of Vita Coco were entitled to payments or product vouchers as benefits in the settlement.

THE BOTTOM LINE

If coconut water actually contains what it is supposed to, then it could be used as a sports drink for shorter-duration sports, but you'd be well advised to look elsewhere if you want to run a marathon or win a day-long soccer tournament. For the rest of us, however, coconut water is still little more than a sugar drink with extra calories that can help expand our waistlines.

SALBA

"Salba—Nature's Healthiest Whole Food" proclaims (sorry, *claimed*) salba.com. The website also stated that, gram for gram, Salba has more antioxidants than blueberries, more calcium than whole milk, more magnesium than broccoli, more fibre than flaxseed, and more omega-3s than salmon. The thing is, the website, which existed when this chapter was first drafted, is gone. For that matter, so is the site salbastore.com, which is where you were redirected to purchase Salba. So what is Salba, why is it trademarked, and why is it so mysterious? Its story is an example of just how complicated things can get in the new world of for-profit superfoods.

SALBA: THE STORY

A product of the *Salvia hispanica* L. plant, Salba is actually a form of chia seed. As the story goes, Argentinian brothers Adolfo and Alfredo Mealla were looking to market chia seeds in the United States, and in the process they approached Dr. Vladimir Vuksan and his team at the University of Toronto St. Michael's Health Centre to inquire about researching the effects of their chia seeds on human health. Upon analyzing the seeds, however, Dr. Vuksan found that the variability in their nutritional value from sample to sample was simply too great to use in clinical trials. So the brothers headed back to Argentina and spent more than a decade cultivating the seeds to produce a more consistent product. By repeatedly growing and sorting the chia seeds, each time replanting the more nutritionally consistent white seeds, the Meallas eventually reached their goal. Ultimately, the new varieties of *Salvia hispanica* L., Sahi Alba (*Alba* means white in Latin) 911 and 912, were given the name Salba, which was then trademarked.[47, 48]

Like chia seeds, Salba can be added to smoothies, yogurt, cereal, or oatmeal. As a high-fibre food, Salba should be introduced to the diet slowly to prevent undesirable side effects, such as gas or bloating, and it should be consumed with plenty of water. Since Salba is a trademarked product, you'll see it in its own distinct packaging—and you won't find it in bulk. Hardly inexpensive at more than a dollar per ounce, a 16-ounce package (providing 24 single-tablespoon servings) of whole-seed Salba sells for $26.99, and a 9-ounce container of ground Salba retails for $19.99.[49]

WILL THE REAL SALBA PLEASE STAND UP?

At the time of writing, the websites salba.com, salbastore.com, and sourcesalba.com were all inactive. Instead, salbasmart.com is currently the place to go for all things Salba, and while at first glance it looks quite different from salba.com, it appears to contain at least a handful of product images, some of which still contain the slogan "Nature's Healthiest Whole Food" that once appeared on salba.com, along with a similar-looking (but not identical) list of nutrient comparisons.[50]

How is this possible for a trademarked food product to exist in two places, seemingly run by two different companies? This mysterious turn of events appears to be the result of legal proceedings launched jointly by Canadian-based Salba Corp. N.A., Colorado's Salba Smart Natural Products (the apparent owner of salbasmart.com), and William A. Ralston and Richard L. Ralston (listed as the managing partner and partner for salbasmart.com) against Florida's X Factor Holdings (which is inactive) and Ancient Naturals. According to the complaint filed by Ralston et al. in 2012, Ancient Naturals was running the now-defunct websites salba.com and salbastore.com, along with salbausa.com and salbarx.com, while engaging in "trademark infringement, trademark counterfeiting, unfair competition, false designation of origin, false advertising, and cyber-squatting."[51] In essence, Ralston et al. accused Ancient Naturals not only of encroaching on their copyright but also of selling Salba that wasn't even Salba. The Ralstons claim they were granted permission to sell the one and only form of pure Salba, imported by the Meallas' own AgriSalba corporation, and that any product sold by rival Ancient Naturals must therefore be a lesser product and, in effect, a fraud.

From digging through court documents, it appears the conflict originated years earlier, when the Mealla brothers minted Salba Research and Development Inc. in 2002 and appointed Toronto resident Lawrence (Larry) Brown as director. According to case files, in 2006, with interest in Salba starting to take off, the Argentinian brothers built a corporation, based out of Toronto and known as Salba Corp. N.A., to hold all the trademarks associated with Salba, and they asked Brown and his sister, Thelma, to serve as figureheads. The Browns were given shares in the company and held some day-to-day responsibilities in running it.[52] The relationship seems to have broken down over time, and by 2009 Lawrence Brown had staked his claim on Salba Corp. N.A., leaving a secondary company, Salba Corp. S.A., to the Meallas. Now in control of a good chunk of the Salba empire, Brown sent a letter to Salba distributors and retailers in 2009 warning that the company they now controlled, Salba Corp. N.A., was "the legal holder of the world-wide trademarks pertaining to 'Salba' and all Salba trademark derivatives" and that they denied the use of the Salba trademark to anyone else, including the Meallas' AgriSalba S.A. and Salba Corp. S.A.[53] It seems the Meallas had been turfed out of their own business by the very people they brought in to help build it.

Around this time, the Meallas were reportedly informed by Mitchell A. Propster that his company, Colorado-based Core Naturals (now Ancient Naturals), would no longer serve as distributor of Salba seeds on their behalf and would instead deal solely with the Browns. Where exactly Ancient Naturals was getting its Salba from wasn't stated in the out-of-court settlement, but the court documents suggest that whatever Core Naturals was selling was not the original Salba obtained from the Meallas.

As you might imagine, the Meallas responded with legal action. In September 2010, they filed a request for an injunction against the Browns, which they were granted,[54] and in May 2012 they filed a complaint, along with the Ralstons, against Ancient Naturals to the U.S. District Court in Colorado.[55] Although a trial date was set for August 2013, the parties advised the court in March 2013 that they had settled the matter out of court, and a four-month stay was granted to ensure the settlement was successfully completed.[56] It is somewhere around this time that all the websites and images related to Ancient Naturals, including salba.com, disappeared, leaving smartsalba.com, operated by the Ralstons, as the place to go for Salba sales and information on the Internet.

SALBA: THE NUTRITION

Since Salba is relatively new to North America, it does not yet appear in the Canadian Nutrient File or the USDA National Nutrient Database, which means that, as with goji and açaí, manufacturers are our main resources for obtaining nutrition information. According to www.salbasmart.com, a 1-tablespoon (15 gram) serving of whole Salba seeds provides 65 calories' worth of energy, along with 3 grams of protein and 5 grams of fibre (the vast majority is insoluble fibre, which is helpful for combatting constipation but might not have much of an effect on cholesterol). Adjusting these numbers to the same serving used for chia and hemp seeds, an ounce (30 grams) of Salba provides 130 calories, a healthy 6 grams of protein, and 10 grams of fibre, rendering it higher in protein than chia but lower than hemp seeds. The fibre is on par with chia. Salba is also naturally gluten free.

While the protein and fibre contents of Salba are significant, what about the other nutrient claims? Well, while salbasmart.com claims it contains "6 x more calcium than whole milk," when you compare realistic serving sizes that an average person would consume, milk contains 290 mg of calcium per cup, versus 116 grams for a tablespoon of Salba. Even if we increase the serving size to 2 tablespoons, or 30 grams, the calcium in Salba is still less than that in a cup of milk and yet would have twice the calories.[57] We also don't yet have published data on how efficiently the calcium from Salba (or chia, for that matter) is absorbed.

Aside from calcium, an ounce of Salba (equal to 2 tablespoons) would provide 12% of your iron needs. Although it is claimed that Salba contains six times more iron than kidney beans, these comparisons are made by weight rather than comparing normal portions that people would actually eat. Likewise, while salbasmart.com boasts that Salba contains twice the potassium of a banana, the 6 tablespoons of Salba you would need in order to reach that level would provide enough fibre (30 grams) that you'd likely spend the rest of your day in the bathroom, and you'd also be on the hook for 390 calories, more than you'll get in a chocolate-covered donut. And yes, at 28% of your daily magnesium, an ounce of Salba contains more magnesium than what you'll get from a cup of broccoli (5%), but broccoli is hardly the standard-bearer in this category. In other words, although the authors of the website technically aren't being untruthful, they are cherry-picking the foods and nutrients they are using for comparison and using unrealistic portions that few people would ever eat.

And what of those omega-3 fatty acid claims? Yes, a 30-gram

serving of Salba offers up a very impressive 6.85 grams of omega-3s, which is higher than both chia and hemp seeds, and on paper it seems to dwarf the 1.5 to 2.5 grams found in 3 ounces of salmon. But the omega-3s are obtained from the plant form of omega-3s, known as alpha-linolenic acid (ALA), which is inefficiently converted to the omega-3 that is most strongly associated with heart health, known as DHA.

SALBA: THE SCIENCE

Perhaps not surprisingly, we have very little research on how Salba affects humans, though Dr. Vuksan's research team did publish two trials (funded by the Mealla brothers) in well-respected medical journals. In one small study, 11 healthy men and women of normal body weight were given 0, 7, 15, or 24 grams of Salba baked into white bread at a single meal, after which blood sugar and appetite ratings were taken for two hours.[58] The researchers found that the more Salba the bread contained, the less of an effect the bread had on blood sugar. The subjects also reported feeling more full on the higher doses of Salba. This at least suggests that, like so many other nuts and seeds, Salba could be an effective tool for controlling blood sugar, and possibly appetite, as long as you consume enough of it: There was no demonstrable benefit from adding Salba at the lower doses.

The second study, a single-blind study published in *Diabetes Care* in 2007, compared the effect of consuming 37 grams of Salba per day versus the same amount of wheat bran over a 12-week period in 20 people with well-controlled type 2 diabetes. Compared with the wheat bran group, those receiving the Salba saw their systolic blood pressure (that's the top number) drop by about 6%, and some measures of blood sugar control improved.[59]

THE BOTTOM LINE

Like most seeds, it's not unreasonable to say that Salba could be a worthy addition to many diets. Rich in protein, fibre, calcium, and magnesium and a source of iron, Salba may well have benefits for blood sugar control, heart health, and appetite control. For now, however, we have limited evidence to back up these assumptions. What we do know is that Salba, like so many superfoods that have big market potential, has run into problems. Remember when going to the grocery store was simple?

POMEGRANATES

For an awfully long time, pomegranate was a fruit that, for many, was more bother than it was worth; that is, until POM Wonderful came along in 2002. Manufacturers of pomegranate juice and juice blends, as well as pomegranate extract pills, POM Wonderful got the world interested in those curious red fruits with the explosive little seeds. Upon hearing claims that pomegranate juice has numerous potential health benefits, ranging from prostate health to heart disease prevention, we all got caught up in the pomegranate hype, at least for a while. As it turns out, however, the cool little superfruit ended up in a bit of hot water.

POMEGRANATES: THE STORY

Pomegranates are believed to be one of the earliest cultivated fruits, with archaeological evidence extending as far back as 3500 B.C. Prominently featured in Greek art, pomegranates are believed to have migrated from Persia to China along the Silk Road around 100 B.C. The Latin name, *Punica granatum*, stems from the fruit's migration through Carthage, North Africa (Carthaginians were known as Punics), while the Latin word *granatum* appropriately describes "many seeds." Pomegranates appear in mythology and historical writings of numerous religions, including Hebrew, Buddhist, and Islamic, and are featured prominently in the Bible. Interestingly, the French term *grenade* is derived from the Latin name for pomegranate, referring to their common shape and capacity to burst into tiny pieces.

Although pomegranates have a long history of use in many parts of the world, POM Wonderful is a more recent phenomenon. Based out of Los Angeles and owned by Lynda and Stewart Resnick, the same billionaire couple who brought us Fiji Water and Teleflora flower delivery, POM Wonderful grows and distributes a specific type of pomegranate, known as the Wonderful.[60] Distinct bulbous bottles, filled with pure or blended pomegranate juice, along with sleek marketing campaigns, helped spur POM Wonderful to sales of US$165 million in 2007.[61] According to the *Chicago Tribune*, the folks at POM Wonderful poured US$34 million into dozens of research studies on the health benefits of pomegranates and pomegranate juices to help bolster their claims.[62]

Unfortunately, things are not as rosy for POM Wonderful today. The problems began in 2010 with a warning letter from the U.S. Food and Drug Administration (FDA), which "found serious violations of the Federal Food, Drug, and Cosmetic Act" on POM Wonderful's website; in essence, the FDA was suggesting that the claims being made by POM Wonderful were consistent with those of a drug. A similar complaint, filed later that same year by the U.S. Federal Trade Commission (FTC), also alleged that POM Wonderful made "false and unsubstantiated" claims in their advertising and on their website, and that the medical research they used to back their claims was flawed.[63] The matter eventually ended up in court, and on May 17, 2012, Chief

Administrative Law Judge D. Michael Chappell issued his initial decision that POM Wonderful had made false or deceptive advertising claims,[64] a decision that was upheld by the FTC eight months later.[65] Specifically, the FTC concluded that 36 of POM Wonderful's ads "deceptively advertised their products and did not have adequate support for claims that the products could treat, prevent, or reduce the risk of heart disease, prostate cancer, and erectile dysfunction, and that they were clinically proven to work."[66] They also ruled that, in the future, POM Wonderful must have two randomized, double-blind, placebo-controlled trials (whenever possible) producing statistically significant effects on valid end points to support their disease claims. In March 2013, POM Wonderful appealed the decision.[67]

POMEGRANATES: THE NUTRITION

Although the science behind POM Wonderful's juices has been disputed, the pomegranate's basic nutritional value has not: A cup (174 grams) of pomegranate arils, or seeds, provides a fairly robust 144 calories, along with 6 grams of fibre. You'll also derive 30% of your vitamin C—not bad, but much less than kiwis and citrus fruits— 36% of your vitamin K, 16% of your folate, and a solid 12% (410 mg) of your potassium for the day. Otherwise, the rest of pomegranate's nutrition profile is simply decent: A cup will give you 8% of your vitamin B_1 and 6% each of your vitamins E, B_2, B_6, and magnesium, as well as 14% of your copper.

POMEGRANATES: THE SCIENCE

What's really unfortunate about the POM Wonderful situation is that, compared with the likes of açaí, noni, and goji, pomegranates have been more extensively studied, often by leading scientists.

However, the FTC ruling against POM Wonderful in 2012 found that many of the 55 studies (some were clinical trials on humans, while others were conducted on animals or on cell lines) funded by the company had design flaws, often lacking blinding (which prevents either the subjects or the researchers, or ideally both, from knowing who is receiving the treatment to reduce the risk of bias) or proper randomizing (where subjects are placed in their treatment group through truly random methods; randomizing reduces bias because it keeps researchers from stacking subjects with certain traits—good or bad—in one group, which could slant their results).

The FTC and the experts who challenged POM Wonderful's research also had concerns about the interpretation of the results POM Wonderful used to fuel its advertising. Much of the dispute stemmed from the use of something known as end points. What is an end point? In the case of heart disease, the main end points are heart attack, strokes, and angina (chest pains)—actual cardiac events. That means if you are studying some type of intervention, be it a dietary change, medication, or supplement, the ultimate measure of its success is how many more people it keeps alive and out of the hospital.

Unfortunately, although testing for end points might be the gold standard for research, as you might imagine, you would need to study an awful lot of people for a very long time to see a significant effect (basically, you have to start the study and then wait for people to get sick or die), a process that is both costly and time consuming and that requires an extremely well-designed and well-controlled study. If it isn't possible to look at end points in a particular study (and it rarely is), then researchers can turn to what are known as surrogate markers, or measures considered to be good predictors of these end points; in the case of heart disease, surrogate markers include HDL ("good") or LDL ("bad") cholesterol, triglycerides, and blood pressure.

Put another way, if your study can't measure death rates or illness, the next best thing is to study the factors that are most closely associated with it. Not all studies look at surrogate markers, however, and therein lies the issue with interpreting their findings: When both end points and surrogates are missing from a study, you need be more cautious when interpreting the results.

Now, back to the POM Wonderful story. In a bit of courtroom drama that saw two research titans go toe to toe, the interpretation of the research of Dr. Michael Aviram at the Technion–Israel Institute, who had previously published some of the seminal studies on red wine and more recently conducted several studies funded by POM Wonderful, was challenged by Dr. Frank Sacks of the Harvard School of Public Health, himself a highly regarded researcher who played a role in developing the well-regarded Dietary Approaches to Stop Hypertension (DASH) diet for controlling blood pressure.

One of the key studies whose results were challenged in court was an often-cited human study out of Dr. Aviram's laboratory, published in the *American Journal of Clinical Nutrition* in 2000, in which 13 healthy male subjects were given 50 ml of pomegranate juice daily for two weeks.[68] Otherwise, the subjects followed their usual dietary routine. At the end of the study, the LDL ("bad" cholesterol) of subjects taking the pomegranate juice wasn't as easily damaged, through a process known as oxidation, and their arteries had less clumping (aggregation) of platelets, a process that starts the buildup of plaques that can ultimately lead to heart attacks.

A second key study from Dr. Aviram's group was published in 2001, this time examining the effects of pomegranate juice on blood pressure.[69] In this study, 10 older adults with high blood pressure were given 50 ml of pomegranate concentrate daily for two weeks. At the end of the study, 7 of the 10 participants saw the activity of something known as angiotensin-converting enzyme, or ACE, drop by an average of 36%, and as a group they saw a statistically significant 5% drop in their systolic blood pressure (the top number). The study concluded that "pomegranate juice consumption can offer a wide protection against cardiovascular disease."

In a rebuttal to Dr. Aviram's research, however, Dr. Sacks testified that, although these and other animal studies conducted by Dr. Aviram's team have some value in allowing us to understand how pomegranates work in the body, the changes to the likes of ACE or platelet aggregation are simply not enough to predict actual heart disease risk for use in advertising a product. In other words, although it's helpful to know that pomegranate juice might reduce ACE (and even then, that is debatable, as this was a small, short-lived study without a control group), that doesn't mean we know it will *actually result in fewer people developing heart disease or dying of a heart attack.* This argument was the core of the FTC's ultimately successful complaint against POM Wonderful.

Aside from the possible effects of pomegranate juice on cardiovascular disease, there is also evidence to suggest it could improve prostate health, reduce inflammation, and improve erectile function. Again, however, the studies used to generate POM Wonderful's many claims were rebutted, one by one, in court.

Although the FTC ruled that POM Wonderful's claims were not substantiated by the research, that didn't mean it was the end of the line for pomegranates. Since the ruling, several other RCTs have been published, with some promising results. In a study examining the effect of pomegranate juice on insulin levels and insulin sensitivity (the ability of the body to effectively "listen" to, or use, insulin to bring blood sugar under control; the disruption of this process is a step on the road to type 2 diabetes), 20 obese adults were given either 120 ml (about 1/2 cup) of pomegranate juice or a placebo daily for a month. Although pomegranate juice came up short when it comes to insulin (it had no effect on either insulin levels or insulin sensitivity), the pomegranate group actually lost more body fat than the control group (increasing by 1.1% in the control group, and decreasing by 1.4% in the pomegranate juice group).[70] Another study, not funded by POM Wonderful, found that pomegranates could help control blood sugar and improve satiety (fullness) by slowing the breakdown of carbohydrates, a process that begins in the mouth.[71] So, it's possible that pomegranates or their juice could play a role in appetite control or weight regulation, but it's far too early to say for sure.

There is also some evidence that pomegranate products could play a role in athletic performance, or more specifically, recovery from it. In one study, conducted at the University of Texas, pomegranate juice was found to improve muscle strength and reduce soreness in the arms (but not in the legs) of 17 men who regularly engaged in weight training.[72] The same research group also found that the muscles of active males who received POMx (pomegranate extract) supplements recovered better after a bout of intense exercise versus placebo.[73] It's not clear how the pomegranate extract worked—there was no difference in levels of inflammation or damage in the muscle—but it at least suggests that pomegranates could be of some benefit to athletes looking to improve their recovery from hard workouts.

HOW TO EAT A POMEGRANATE

Despite all their controversy, pomegranates are still delicious and quite good for you. The trick, however, is to get the seeds out without wearing them. To do this, simply cut off the top of the pomegranate, then make a series of thin slices that go just through the skin from top to bottom (almost like slicing an orange). Looking at it from the top, the pomegranate does have natural segments separated by white webbing, known as pith—use the webbing as your guide. Soak the pomegranate in water for a few minutes to soften the peel, and then pull off the skin and separate the pith from the seeds. Voila! Pomegranate seeds without the grenade-like effect.

THE BOTTOM LINE

How did a simple fruit become so complicated? It almost boggles the mind that the question of whether or not a pomegranate or its juice is good for you ended up in court, but that's the way it goes in the complicated world of marketing superfoods. Pomegranates are nutritious; no one is disputing that. But will drinking their juice keep you from having a heart attack, protect you from prostate cancer, or help you be a better athlete? That is far less clear. In the meantime, POM juices still sit on store shelves—albeit with much less fanfare for now—while POM Wonderful funds the clinical trials that will meet the court-decreed standards for health claims in advertising. Only time will tell how this story ends.

2

QUINOA, I THOUGHT
I KNEW YA

SUPERFOODS WITH QUESTION MARKS

Although some superfoods have checkered pasts, others have raised eyebrows for different reasons. Recently, quinoa has been in the headlines, for example, because of concerns that the booming quinoa industry is hurting the same Bolivians who produce it. Agave, on the other hand, is the subject of hot debate because of concerns that it contains a potentially harmful type of sugar. And hemp seeds? They're still illegal to grow in the United States.

In an Internet era, where the 24-hour news cycle has devolved into 20 minutes of Tweets, our desire to anoint the latest, greatest superfood means we don't take much time to figure out if it has any real merit—or potential drawbacks—before we run it up the flagpole. As a result, although we might be having a love affair with chia, coconut, hemp, and even—yawn—quinoa, the question still lingers: What evidence do we really have that these foods are as good for us as we might believe? The answer? Not much, and yet their popularity endures.

QUINOA

If oats and broccoli were the original superfoods, quinoa was their love child. Virtually unheard of in North America a decade ago, quinoa's rise to prominence began when a NASA-commissioned study dubbed it suitable for use in long-term human space missions.[1] Renowned for its protein content, which includes all nine essential amino acids—a rarity in plants—quinoa has, in the last decade, emerged from fringe health food to supermarket mainstay and has triggered dozens of product spinoffs and even entire cookbooks in the process.[2] Quinoa's rise in global popularity has reached such proportions that the United Nations' Food and Agriculture Organization (FAO) went so far as to dub 2013 "the International Year of Quinoa."

Unfortunately, quinoa's rise to popularity has been accompanied by accusations that its eager adoption by health-conscious Western-ers is causing unintended and undesirable consequences for quinoa growers in South America, making it something of a case study in the effects of rapid spikes in consumption triggered by the superfood trend. So what, exactly, makes quinoa so special, and does the truth match the hype? And how real are the social and environmental con-sequences associated with its rapid rise in popularity?

QUINOA: THE STORY

Quinoa (pronounced KEEN-wah) is often mislabelled as a grain. More accurately, it is a pseudocereal or pseudograin, since it is derived from a seed plant rather than from grasses, such as oats or wheat. Quinoa is actually part of the same ecological goosefoot family as beets, spinach, and Swiss chard—not exactly the company you would expect to keep if you were a traditional grain.

Grown largely in South America, quinoa has seen its production hub shift in recent years from Peru to Bolivia, the latter of which is now responsible for an estimated 46% of the world's quinoa production. Quinoa has reportedly been cultivated in the Altiplano, the high plains of the Andes Mountains, for more than 5,000 years; it is a rare plant that tolerates dry, arid land.

QUINOA: THE NUTRITION

Nutritionally, quinoa has much to offer: A cup of cooked quinoa provides 222 calories, along with 5 grams of fibre and as much protein as a cup of milk (8 grams). It is also a source of more than 10% of your daily needs for several B vitamins (B_1, B_2, B_6, and folate), along with an impressive complement of minerals, including 15% of your iron, 30% of your magnesium, and 13% of your zinc requirements for a day. In particular, its iron and zinc content are unusually high for a plant food, and that, along with a full complement of essential protein-building amino acids, including lysine (an uncommon amino acid in plant foods), makes it a popular choice for those on plant-based diets.

Although data from the Canadian Nutrient File and the USDA National Nutrient Database might leave you with the impression you can reliably predict just how nutritious quinoa is, the reality is there are many different cultivars, or types, of quinoa being grown, and nutritional composition, including the amount of protein and proportion of amino acids, can vary from one to the next.[3] More concerning is the fact that, although quinoa is generally considered a gluten-free food, a 2012 study of 15 different cultivars found that two had the potential to trigger a response for those with celiac disease.[4] Since the research was the first of its kind, further studies are clearly needed.

QUINOA: THE SCIENCE

For all the hype surrounding quinoa, you would expect that it be backed by at least a handful of high-quality human studies. In fact, the research conducted to date relates mostly to its nutritional content or its theoretical potential (as yet untested and unproven) to prevent or manage medical conditions, such as diabetes, heart disease, or celiac disease. We do know that quinoa has a low glycemic index (GI) (cooked quinoa has a GI of 53, compared with 100 for pure glucose sugar), which means it doesn't tend to cause big spikes in blood sugar. Otherwise, no studies have been conducted comparing the effects of eating quinoa versus other grains, seeds, or any food for that matter, on any outcome—including weight, blood sugar or cholesterol control, overall nutritional status, or disease risk.

COOKING WITH QUINOA

No doubt, one of quinoa's great assets is its versatility. It is most commonly prepared and used in much the same way as rice or couscous: simmered in water or stock until fluffy and tender, then served as a side dish, with or without chopped veggies, herbs, spices, or even fruit (cranberries, raisins, and dried apricots complement quinoa particularly well). Quinoa flakes can be made into a breakfast cereal, much like oatmeal, or used in baking. Quinoa can also be ground into flour that can be used in lieu of wheat flour, although the occasionally coarser texture may not be suitable in all recipes. Quinoa seeds can be soaked and sprouted, making them an option for raw-food enthusiasts.

Several different colours of quinoa are available on the market. White or golden quinoa is most common, but red and black quinoa are becoming more popular. Roughly speaking, all types of quinoa may be used interchangeably in cooking, but the nutritional value will vary between colours and brands.

When cooking with quinoa, it is recommended that you start by rinsing or soaking the seeds to minimize the taste of saponins, the bitter, soap-like compounds that serve as a natural protective barrier against insects and other pests. Although most saponins are mechanically removed during processing, one extra rinse can help ensure optimal taste.

CONSEQUENCES OF CONSUMPTION

The vast increase in demand for quinoa is rapidly changing the face of its production and marketing. According to the FAO, Bolivian quinoa production increased from just over 20,000 metric tons in 2000 to 38,000 metric tons in 2011, and land use for quinoa increased by more than 50% in that time.[5] Although much of Bolivia's quinoa is used domestically, the international appetite for quinoa has fueled an export market, mostly to the United States and Europe, worth nearly US$85 million. Perhaps it is not surprising, then, that the price of quinoa almost tripled on the international market in just five years, rising from US$1,150 per ton in 2006 to US$3,115 in 2011.[6]

As a result of this rapid rise in popularity, countries such as Bolivia are racing to catch up to the demand, and the fallout has raised some concern. Ecologically, it is said that cultivating mass amounts of quinoa without allowing fallow years, or those in which the seed is not harvested, can lead to depletion of soil quality and a rise in desert-like conditions. Llama guano—or poop, for the less politically correct— serves as a natural fertilizer for quinoa, and there have been reports that llama herds have been declining as the demand for growing space for quinoa rises. *Time* magazine,[7] the *New York Times*,[8] and National Public Radio[9] in the United States have all recently run stories on the potential concerns associated with quinoa farming, highlighting at-times violent land disputes and the difficulty native Bolivians are experiencing in affording quinoa because of rising costs.

Several groups working directly with Bolivian farmers, however, including the filmmaking team of Stefan Jeremiah and Michael Wilcox, who celebrate the FAO's declaration of 2013 as "the International Year of Quinoa" in their upcoming documentary *The Mother Grain*, counter that these reports are misguided and sensationalist. Jeremiah and Wilcox have made several trips to Bolivia and have spent considerable time with Bolivian farmers growing quinoa. The filmmakers claim that the farming community in Bolivia has benefited significantly from quinoa's rise in popularity, allowing those from once-impoverished regions the opportunity to afford fresh fruits, vegetables, and meats and to improve access to education for their children. In an interview I conducted with Jeremiah for my *National Post* column, he says the claims that quinoa has been outpriced for the average Bolivian are inaccurate. In fact, he said, quinoa is traditionally seen as a poor man's food. "The people like you and me don't eat quinoa," said Jeremiah. "It's passé, it's old school, it's not on their radar." Unfortunately, in Jeremiah's eyes, this negative press could unfairly harm quinoa's reputation on the international market, with downstream economic consequences that could be detrimental to Bolivians. "The media have picked up on something that is trivial and sensationalized it—and that is going to hurt the farmers."

Now, you might ask the question, why not grow it ourselves? Although there have been efforts to expand quinoa's growing territory into other high-altitude regions in Canada and the United States, Jeremiah claims that Bolivian scientists, who worked with NASA on the early studies on quinoa's special nutrition profile, have found that much of quinoa's broad spectrum of nutrients is derived from the close growing proximity to the nutrient-rich Salar de Uyuni, or salt plains, of the Altiplano region of the Andes Mountains. It is the minerals in these salts that make quinoa so nutritious, which means that quinoa grown in other parts of the world might not have the same value. Of course, we need more research to know whether or not these claims are true.

THE BOTTOM LINE

Quinoa, in many ways, is the quintessential superfood: richly nutritious (at least on paper) and poorly understood. Despite this lack of understanding of its actual health benefits, our desire to tap into foods with the highest-possible nutrition profile means that quinoa's popularity has taken off like a rocket, but with that could well come social and ecological consequences that reach far beyond our dinner plates.

CHIA SEEDS

Chia seeds are the seeds of the *Salvia hispanica* L. plant, and if you're old enough, you might have used them to grow a Chia Pet in the 1970s or '80s. Yes, it's true: The same chia seeds that were supposed to keep kids happy enough that they wouldn't ask for a real pet are now hot stuff in the nutrition world. And although the Chia Pet is still alive and well (in fact, Joseph Enterprises, the makers of the Chia Pet and other made-for-TV products with fabulous jingles, including the Clapper and the 'Ove' Glove, have expanded their chia offerings to now include Chia Hello Kitty, Chia SpongeBob, and Chia Bart Simpson),[10] it is the dark grey seeds that are spread on the terracotta figurines that have been the focus of much recent interest.

CHIA SEEDS: THE STORY

Chia is a member of the mint family, and despite appearances, it can grow to a full 3 feet (1 metre) tall, eventually producing large white or purple flowers. Its seeds are said to have been dubbed "chia" by the Aztecs and other pre-Columbian societies, who used it therapeutically. Originally cultivated in Mexico, Guatemala, and other parts of South and Central America, chia is now grown in Australia and Southeast Asia, where it is known for its ability to tolerate suboptimal conditions, including dry spells, making it a popular crop for sustainable development.

CHIA SEEDS: THE NUTRITION

A 1-ounce serving of dried chia seeds provides about 137 calories' worth of energy, which makes it one of the lowest-calorie foods from the nut and seed family. Compared with hemp seeds, chia seeds are lower in protein (4 grams versus 10 grams per ounce) but higher in fibre (11 grams versus 3 grams per ounce), and they provide twice the ALA (that's the plant form of omega-3 fat), at 5 grams per ounce. Unfortunately, even that large quantity of ALA seems to have limited impact on the body's ability to produce DHA, the omega-3 fatty acid thought to have the biggest impact on our health, especially when it comes to our hearts. In a study published in the journal *Plant Foods and Human Nutrition*, U.S. researchers found that although post-menopausal women given 25 grams of milled chia seeds per day for seven weeks saw an increase in their circulating levels of ALA and EPA (another omega-3 fatty acid), there was no change in their DHA levels.[11] Several studies have demonstrated that animals fed chia seeds produce meat or eggs with higher omega-3 fatty acid content than those fed flaxseed or canola/rapeseed.[12] Once again, however, the omega-3 increase is attributable to ALA, rather than DHA, making it difficult to say if this will translate to any significant clinical benefit for humans.

Interestingly, not all chia seeds are made equal: As chia seeds mature, their omega-3 (ALA) content drops, while the amount of omega-6 fatty acids, known as linoleic acid, rises.[13] Likewise, chia grown at higher altitudes and in cooler temperatures seems to have relatively more polyunsaturated fatty acids (or PUFAs, the family of fats that includes omega-3 and omega-6 fatty acids), while chia grown in warmer, lower-altitude environments is richer in saturated fat. In theory, then, the best chia seeds would be grown at altitude and harvested young: Those growing conditions would give consumers the most omega-3 and the least saturated fat. Unfortunately, this information is rarely available to consumers, so this recommendation is basically an academic one.

Chia seeds are gluten free, making them a logical choice for those with celiac disease and non-celiac gluten sensitivity. Like so many other foods that have only recently gained popularity in the Western diet, however, we don't yet have a complete picture of chia's nutritional value. Although we do know that chia appears to be a remarkably good source of calcium, providing about 177 mg per ounce, or about 20% of a healthy adult's daily needs, we really can't say much about chia's other nutrients at this point, including iron, selenium, magnesium, and vitamin E content, all of which are typically present in nuts and seeds. In other words, there is a lot of hype about chia's nutrition, but it isn't based on a whole lot of substance.

CHIA SEEDS: THE SCIENCE

In animal studies, feeding chia to rats has resulted in reduced levels of LDL cholesterol, as well as triglycerides, a type of fat in the bloodstream associated with heart disease. HDL, or the so-called good cholesterol, tends to rise.[14] The results in humans, however, have been much less impressive. In one study, subjects with metabolic syndrome (a cluster of symptoms, such as high-normal blood sugars, high triglycerides, and a larger-than-ideal waist circumference, which is associated with an increased risk of developing type 2 diabetes and heart disease) who took a chia-containing drink for three months did see their triglycerides and C-reactive protein (a measure of inflammation in the body) drop significantly compared with a placebo drink.[15] Unfortunately, because the drink contained a combination of known cholesterol-lowering foods, including soy protein, oats, and nopal (a popular Mexican food derived from prickly pear), we don't know how much of the effect the chia seeds had on their own.

Fortunately, a group of researchers at Appalachian State University have looked specifically at the impact of eating chia, both as a seed and milled as a flour, on various measures related to weight and heart health, but the results haven't exactly been overwhelming. In their first study, the researchers gave a group of otherwise healthy overweight and obese men and women 25 grams of chia twice per day and compared those results with a placebo.[16] After three months, the chia had no effect on blood pressure, inflammation, or oxidative stress (damage on a cellular level as a result of aging, pollution, and poor diet that is thought to contribute to heart disease and cancer risk). Chia also had no effect on weight or body composition (either by reducing body fat or increasing muscle mass or both) versus a placebo.

In a second study, the same team gave 25 grams of milled or whole chia seeds per day to a group of overweight women. After 10 weeks, the subjects taking the milled chia seeds had higher circulating levels of ALA and EPA, but interestingly, the same was not true for those taking whole chia seeds. Perhaps it's the case, then, that the whole chia seed is hard enough to digest that our bodies struggle to extract all the key nutrients, as is also the case with flaxseed. When it came down to the other outcomes measured in the study, however, the type of chia didn't seem to matter: There was no difference in body composition, inflammation, or blood pressure between the milled and whole chia seed group—and no difference compared with a placebo, either.[17] So, if chia does have a measurable effect on health or weight, it seems you'll either need to take it for a prolonged period of time or you'll have to take a fairly high dose to get there.

Aside from examining overweight or obese individuals, at least one study has looked at the impact of giving chia to athletes. In a study on young, healthy male runners, researchers found that drinking a combination of a chia-based drink and Gatorade was just as effective as drinking Gatorade alone when it came to preparing for a long (90 minute-plus) run.[18] This isn't an entirely surprising finding, since chia is a relatively good source of energy-providing carbohydrates, as is a sports drink. On the other hand, chia is also more nutritious than a traditional sports drink, which could make it a popular choice among health-conscious athletes. Before you toss your Gatorade in favour of chia drinks, however, be warned: Chia is very high in fibre, and that can mean digestive upset (read: bloating, gas, nausea, cramping, and even diarrhea) for athletes, especially in high-intensity and endurance activities. The bottom line: One study is not enough to put chia on the list of "best sports drinks" for athletic performance, but it at least suggests that more research is warranted.

EATING CHIA

If you haven't tried chia before, prepare yourself for something a little different. Unlike most nuts and seeds, chia absorbs considerable water, making oatmeal, yogurt, and smoothies thicker, especially if you add the chia a few minutes before eating. This gel-like quality means chia can be used in vegetarian and vegan recipes as an egg substitute or for puddings. Unlike eggs, however, chia will not help baked goods rise. Although chia is becoming more widely known, it is still mostly available in health and bulk food stores, where it can be quite expensive, often reaching around $10 for a 12-ounce (340 gram) package. Fortunately, chia works well in smaller portions: 1 to 3 tablespoons is enough for most people.

THE BOTTOM LINE

Despite its surge in popularity, it is still early days for chia seeds, at least if you're interested in facts and evidence. Although the nutrition profile of this South American seed suggests it may be valuable for cholesterol and blood sugar control, not to mention bowel health, the research to date simply hasn't panned out. With a capacity to grow in arid environments, chia could be an important crop in the new green economy, but questions about the variations in its nutrient composition when grown in different conditions still need to be answered. Overall, chia can be enjoyed fairly freely, including by those on gluten-free diets, and serves as a good alternative and complement to hemp and flaxseed. As for its superfood status? It's simply too early to say for sure.

HEMP SEEDS

Hemp seeds are a product of the *Cannabis sativa* plant, but they are not the same strain of hemp as the stuff Bill Clinton never inhaled. Touted for its protein and omega-3 fatty acid content, hemp and its products, including whole hemp seeds and their hulled hearts (hemp hearts) have made the leap from fringe product to the nutrition mainstream and can now be found, along with hemp protein powder, hemp oil, and other hemp-derived products, in health food stores and mainstream grocery stores alike.

HEMP SEEDS: THE STORY

Hemp has a prolonged history of use by humans, dating back some 10,000 years. In China, it was used not only for food but also as a commodity, to make rope, cloth, sails, and even paper, and that versatility of use continued in many parts of the world until the 20th century. Through the 1700s and 1800s, hemp was said to light Abraham Lincoln's home and serve as paper for draft versions of the U.S. Declaration of Independence (you may have heard that the Constitution, Declaration of Independence, and Bill of Rights were written on hemp, but constitutional experts claim that, although the drafts may have used hemp paper, which was common at the time, the final versions were actually written on parchment paper).[19] The U.S. Department of Agriculture even launched a "Hemp for Victory" program during the Second World War, encouraging U.S. farmers to help the government increase hemp production to support the war movement.[20]

Despite hemp's long history of multi-purpose use, the Controlled Substances Act of 1970 eventually deemed it illegal to grow in the United States (it was already illegal to possess in many states), and that is how it remains to this day—that is, unless you can get the Drug Enforcement Administration (DEA) to give you permission to grow it.[21] As recently as 2001, the DEA sought to ban the sale of hemp foods in the United States, a decision that triggered a three-year battle with the Hemp Industries Association, ultimately culminating with the Ninth U.S. Circuit Court of Appeals ruling against the DEA. The bottom line? Although it is legal to sell and distribute hemp in the United States, it is still not legal to grow it.[22]

In Canada, farmers were encouraged to grow hemp in the 1920s, which was used, among other things, for oil. Nevertheless, hemp was banned, along with marijuana, in Canada in 1938, a year after the Marihuana Tax Act was introduced in the United States. In the 1990s, however, hemp resurfaced in Manitoba, where research demonstrated that it can be grown without any detectable levels of THC (tetra-hydrocannabinol), the opioid compound responsible for marijuana's "high." By 1998, hemp was legalized in Canada, and its profile, both as a food and as a commodity, has been on the rise ever since.[23]

HEMP SEEDS: THE NUTRITION

Because they are relatively new to the mass market, much of the nutrition information on hemp hearts is supplied by the industry. According to Manitoba Harvest Hemp Foods, producers of hemp-based products in Canada, a 1-ounce (30 gram) or 3-tablespoon serving of hemp hearts provides 170 calories' worth of energy, along with 10 grams of protein. Of the 13 grams of fat in a serving of hemp hearts, about 2.5 grams are derived from omega-3 fatty acids in the plant-based form, ALA. Much of the remainder (about 60% of the fat content) is derived from omega-6 fats, including linoleic acid, as well as a type of fat known as gamma-linoleic acid, or GLA (more on that later). This provides hemp seeds with an intriguing ratio of omega-6 to omega-3 of about 3.5:1, which is within the range that some experts consider "optimal" for human health (see the sidebar The Great Omega-6:Omega-3 Debate for more). A serving of hemp hearts also contains 3 grams of fibre, has 1 gram of sugar, and is naturally gluten free.

When it comes to vitamins and minerals, hemp hearts stand out for their zinc and magnesium content, providing 30% of your daily zinc needs and a whopping 70% of your magnesium requirements in a 3-tablespoon serving. Magnesium is a vital nutrient that is often underconsumed in the North American diet, yet it plays an important role in health, so the potential contribution of hemp to our magnesium intake should not be overlooked. A recent review on magnesium for heart health, for example, using data from previous studies, suggested that low levels of magnesium in the diet may be associated with increased risk factors for cardiovascular disease, including inflammation in the arteries, a higher level of C-reactive protein (a measure of inflammation in all parts of the body), and endothelial dysfunction (damaged arteries).[24] Since magnesium is largely available in nuts, seeds, and whole grains, however, it's necessary to eat a well-balanced, high-quality diet to meet your needs; perhaps it's not surprising, then, that more than one-third of Canadian adults don't get enough magnesium in their diets.[25]

As for hemp's zinc content, since plant foods tend to be lower in this all-important mineral for wound healing, healthy skin, and a strong immune system, foods such as hemp hearts can be particularly valuable for vegetarians or those who eat less animal protein in their diets. Hemp could also be a useful addition to the diet of older adults, who are also prone to missing their dietary targets for zinc.

The nutritional value of hemp seeds doesn't end with magnesium and zinc, however: A 30-gram serving also boasts a solid 30% of your iron and thiamin (vitamin B_1), 10% of your vitamin B_6, and 15% of your folate, as well as a whole day's manganese (which, to be fair, is a very common nutrient in many foods).

THE GREAT OMEGA-6:OMEGA-3 DEBATE

There is a long-standing theory that, although omega-6 fatty acids are essential to human health, the Western diet is simply too rich in them. Omega-6 is commonly consumed through vegetable oils such as corn, sunflower, and safflower oils and in margarines, dressings, baked goods, and processed foods, but there is concern that excessive amounts contribute to inflammation in the body, effectively "drowning out" the beneficial anti-inflammatory effects of omega-3 fatty acids. Although our current diet is estimated to provide a whole lot more omega-6s than omega-3s (perhaps about 15 to 17 times more omega-6 than omega-3),[26] early humans likely ate a ratio closer to 4:1 or even less.[27] As a result, there is a sense that increasing the omega-3 fats in our diets, while also reducing our reliance on processed foods rich in omega-6, could improve our health, especially as it relates to diseases of inflammation in the heart, brain, joints, and virtually every other part of our bodies.[28]

On the other hand, current dietary guidelines for both Canada and the United States recommend increasing polyunsaturated fats from *both* sources—omega-3 and omega-6—in place of saturated fats, the solid fats at room temperature that include butter, fatty cuts of red meat, full-fat dairy products, and coconut and palm oil.[29] These guidelines are based on research suggesting that reducing saturated fats and replacing them with either type of PUFA is beneficial for our cholesterol and overall risk of heart disease. This debate has been raging for years, and it became even more contentious with more recent research suggesting that saturated fats may not be as harmful as we once thought. In reality, the effect of altering the omega-6 to omega-3 ratio is not black and white, and even very recent studies have been contradictory.[30] The bottom line? Whether or not hemp seed's ratio of omega-6 to omega-3 is worthy of bragging rights remains to be determined.

HEMP SEEDS: THE SCIENCE

So far, hemp products might sound almost too good to be true: nutritionally rich, seemingly good for the environment, and easy to add to common foods, such as oatmeal or smoothies. For all of this promise, however, we actually know little about how hemp functions in humans.

On a theoretical level, hemp's fat and fibre content should probably be good for your heart. True to form, an extract taken from hemp seed prevented damage to LDL ("bad") cholesterol better than extracts from other presumed-to-be heart-healthy foods, such as flaxseed, grape seed, and soybean extracts, at least in a test tube.[31] Hemp seed meal has also showed promise in the treatment of high cholesterol and cardiovascular disease as well as Alzheimer's disease (but not Parkinson's or Huntington's disease)—in fruit flies.[32] If you want to keep rats healthy, 12 weeks on a diet rich in hemp seed can help repair their heart tissue after a heart attack or other injury,[33] while a diet made up of 10% hemp seed (equivalent to about 200 calories, or just over 3 tablespoons per day for an average adult) reduces platelet aggregation, a starting point in the formation of a plaque in the arteries, in rabbits.[34] Finally, if you have aging rodents at home, you might be pleased to know that a diet of up to 10% hemp seed for three weeks appears to reduce complications associated with menopause, both by controlling cholesterol levels and by reducing feelings of anxiety.[35]

On the other hand, human research on hemp seed is almost non-existent. In one of the only human trials to date, Finnish researchers compared hemp seed oil versus olive oil for the treatment of eczema (atopic dermatitis). In this 20-week single-blind study (meaning the subjects were unaware of which treatment they were receiving, but the researchers were aware), hemp seed oil decreased water loss from the skin, improved skin dryness, and reduced itchiness while reducing the need for medication.[36] Hemp seed's potential to improve skin health might be attributable to its gamma-linoleic acid (GLA) content, a type of omega-6 fatty acid involved with skin lubrication that individuals with eczema tend to lack (GLA is also found in borage oil and evening primrose oil). To date, however, that is about all we know about hemp's effects in humans.

CONSEQUENCES OF CONSUMPTION

Dubbed "the world's premier renewable resource" in a report published by Agriculture and Agri-Food Canada, hemp has huge potential to help a strained environment.[37] With the ability to transform into clothing, food, paper, oil, cosmetics, paints, and even beer, hemp's potential to become a source for more sustainable building materials, including insulation, carpeting, and paneling, is being explored. Hemp is even strong enough that it could be used for automotive parts (it is even said that Henry Ford built a car using hemp products).

Manitoba Harvest Hemp Foods, whose mission is to be the world's leader in the production and distribution of hemp food products, claims to be the world's only vertically integrated hemp food company. That means it controls every aspect of the process of growing and distributing its product, and it partners with hemp farmers to produce a product that is both high quality and kind to Earth. All the ingredients are organic and fair-traded, and the company offsets all its production facility's electricity and natural gas usage with renewable energy credits and carbon offsets. Manitoba Harvest claims the impact of its conservation has been the equivalent of planting 1,009 mature trees, or not driving 272,449 miles in an average car.

THE BOTTOM LINE

After nearly a century on the outs, hemp and its associated foods have made up a lot of ground in a relatively short time. Although hemp's protein and magnesium content are exceptional, its potential as a renewable resource is also worthy of our attention. But—there's always a but—we have to bear in mind that the research on hemp's health benefits is virtually non-existent in humans, so for now, we are taking something of a leap of faith by assuming its nutrition profile will translate into meaningful outcomes. Only time will tell.

COCONUT

If there's one controversial superfood that has enjoyed a transition into the mainstream, it's probably coconut oil. It has long been reviled for its exceptionally high saturated fat content, but a greater understanding of the way the fats in coconut are metabolized has led some medical and nutrition experts to lean in the direction that the alternative health community has for years: Namely, that coconut might not only be okay for heart health but could actually be good for us. But that doesn't mean everyone is in agreement: In many corners, coconut is still viewed as a potential trigger for heart disease that should be strictly avoided.

COCONUT: THE STORY

Coconut (*Cocos nucifera*) is a tropical fruit that is commonly consumed in equatorial nations, including Malaysia, Indonesia, Thailand, and the Philippines. It is believed that coconuts spread by floating from island to island throughout Asia and the South Pacific. On land, coconut palm trees usually grow in low-lying areas, near the high-water mark where there is plenty of rain and groundwater. A single tree can produce 50 to 100 coconuts per year, which can be put to numerous uses, both edible and non-edible: Its husk, for example, can be used to make a fibre known as coir, which can be used to make textiles such as mats, rope, and baskets and is highly sought after by gardeners who use it to line planters and hanging baskets.[38]

COCONUT: THE NUTRITION

Coconut can be eaten several ways: as raw coconut meat (usually shredded and added as an ingredient to other foods), as coconut milk (grated coconut meat in water), and as coconut oil.

Coconut Meat

If you prefer your coconut straight up, you're in for 283 calories per cup, shredded. Compared with a cup of most fruits and vegetables, that is an awful lot of calories and would probably feel pretty heavy because of its high fat content. More reasonably, a 2-inch-by-2-inch chunk of coconut, which weighs in at about 1.5 ounces, or 45 grams—picture something a bit smaller than the average chocolate bar—provides a slightly more svelte 159 calories, along with 15 grams of fat (13 of which are saturated, the so-called bad fat, but more on that in a moment), 4 grams of fibre, and 3 grams of sugar. Protein is the least represented macronutrient in coconut, with only 1 gram in a 45-gram serving.

Nutritionally, 45 grams of coconut will provide 6% of your iron (1.1 mg), 5% of your phosphorus, 5% of your potassium (160 mg), 6% of your selenium, and 10% of your copper for the day. These are certainly better-than-nothing numbers, but they aren't exactly screaming superfood, either. In other words, if you're eating coconut, it's not so much for the vitamins and minerals, unless you're into eating whole coconuts at once.

Coconut Milk

Coconut milk differs from coconut water in that both the meat and the water are used, yielding a thicker, denser, and therefore higher-calorie product than coconut water. A cup of canned coconut milk provides 445 calories—yes, that's right—along with 48 grams of fat, of which 43 are saturated. Put another way, a cup of coconut milk provides about three times the calories you'll find in a can of pop, or about the same as a medium order of fries. Unlike so many junk foods, however, coconut milk will at least give you a load of nutrients for your 400-plus calories, including 5 grams of protein, 41% of your daily iron, 26% of your magnesium, 14% (497 mg) of your potassium, 8% of your zinc and folate, and 7% of your niacin (vitamin B_3) needs for the day. Well, if you're going to eat about as many calories as there are in a Big Mac, at least you're going to get something worthwhile out of it . . .

Coconut Oil

Finally, there is coconut oil: that distinctive-tasting creamy, white oil that was once banished for heart health but is now making a comeback as both a supplement and as an ingredient. Like all oils, coconut oil is high in calories: A tablespoon (14 grams/15 ml) provides 116 calories, essentially the same as a tablespoon of olive oil (119 calories). All the calories come via 14 grams of fat, of which a whopping 12 grams are saturated—that's 60% of the so-called bad fat most healthy people are supposed to eat in a day. Otherwise, coconut oil, like most oils, offers no vitamins, minerals, fibre, or protein.

Now, this is where it gets more complicated: Although coconut oil is rich in saturated fat, it is not the same kind of saturated fat you'll find in animal fats. Made up primarily of 12- and 14-carbon-long fats known as lauric acid and myristic acid, the fats in coconut are known as medium-chain triglycerides, or MCTs. Comparatively, the saturated fats that are most widely associated (and even then, debatably so) with high cholesterol and heart disease are 16 carbons and longer, known scientifically as long-chain fatty acids, or LCFAs. MCTs, as it turns out, are metabolized differently from LCFAs, by entering the bloodstream and immediately becoming available as an energy source, whereas LCFAs are repackaged in the liver and can eventually be taken up by our body's fat stores. It's this fundamental difference in metabolism that could explain some of the unexpected effects of coconut oil versus other saturated fats.

COCONUT: THE SCIENCE

Some fascinating research has been published on populations that consume coconut on a regular basis. In a classic study, published in the *American Journal of Clinical Nutrition* in 1981, Dr. Ian Prior and associates undertook a detailed analysis of the diets of two Polynesian populations: the Pukapuka and Tokelau.[39] Over the course of the study, which started in 1964 with the Pukapuka and continued with both groups though the mid-1970s, the two populations were still largely isolated from contact by the developed world. Other than the occasional cargo ship providing canned meat, rice, and preserved foods, both Polynesian groups still consumed their traditional diets, which largely consisted of coconut, starchy vegetables (either taro or breadfruit), and fish. Chicken and pork were eaten occasionally at celebrations, but eggs were not consumed. The main difference between the two diets was that the Pukapuka consumed cereal grains, making up about 30% of their daily calories (notably, their triglycerides were also higher, which we commonly see when carbohydrate foods, such as cereal grains, increase in the diet), while the Tokelau consumed none.

The real story, however, was their collective coconut intake, which was astounding: Coconuts made up 34% of total energy for the Pukapuka and 63%—yes, 63%—of daily calories (not just fat) for the Tokelau. Based on their estimated caloric intakes, that translates to about 1,500 calories' worth of coconut per day for the Tokelau. So, if the theory that coconut is bad for your heart holds water, then surely a group with an intake that high should have been dropping like flies from heart disease and strokes, even if they didn't partake in the other heart-unhealthy habits of the industrialized world. As you might have guessed, however, that simply was not the case; in both groups, heart disease was virtually non-existent—that is, until they moved to New Zealand and abandoned their traditional ways. (Another interesting wrinkle to this story is that neither group consumed any significant amount of green vegetables; instead, they derived virtually all their nutrition from the three or four nutrient-dense foods already mentioned.)

Of course, anyone with a critical eye will point out that many factors likely contributed to the healthy hearts of these Polynesian populations. They didn't smoke, didn't drink, and had a lifestyle free of remote controls and laptops. Of course, genetics might have also been a factor. Fair enough, but a study such as this is in many ways a relatively well-controlled one because it has so few variables: basically, that a diet consisting of only a handful of foods, including an almost absurd amount of coconut, would allow a population to exist for so long.

Coconut and Heart Health

Although population studies give us a good starting point for further research, they can prove only correlation between coconut and health, not causation. So what do we have in the way of well-controlled studies on coconut intake? Here, we see some interesting and yet conflicting results: On the one hand, it seems that eating coconut triggers an increase in cholesterol levels, especially LDL cholesterol,[40, 41] and on the other, population studies suggest that coconut is *not* associated with heart disease risk.[42, 43, 44] Part of the explanation for coconut's seemingly conflicting effects could be related to its effect on HDL, or good, cholesterol: While LDL does drift northward when coconut is consumed, the same is true for HDL, which also tends to climb with coconut intake.[45, 46]

A slightly older but still intriguing study gives a deeper understanding of coconut's effects compared with other fats. The study used margarines that were either high or low in saturated fat from coconut oil (in the low saturated fat arm of the study, the saturated fats were replaced with carbohydrates) as well as a margarine with equal calories but high in unsaturated fats (the family of fats considered the most heart-healthy). The women who took the coconut oil–based margarine that was high in saturated fat saw their total cholesterol climb moderately (from an average of 4.95 to 5.38 mmol/L), as did their LDL cholesterol (from 2.99 to 3.20 mmol/L), over the course of the study.[47] Their HDL cholesterol, however—remember, that's the so-called good cholesterol—also rose from 1.42 to 1.69 mmol/L, and an important marker of the healthiest kind of HDL, known as apolipoprotein A-1, was higher in the coconut oil group than any other group. Perhaps most intriguingly, while the LDL of the coconut oil group did rise, their levels of apolipoprotein B, a marker of small, dense LDL—considered the worst kind of LDL cholesterol—didn't.

So how did the other groups fare? The high-unsaturated-fat group significantly improved their total and LDL cholesterol, and unlike the coconut oil group, their apoB levels actually dropped. In contrast to the coconut oil group, however, their HDL and apoA-1 were unchanged—in other words, while the unsaturated fat group came out better in the "bad" cholesterol measures, the coconut oil group ruled the day on the "good" cholesterol side of things. Ironically, the group that came out looking the worst was the one given the low saturated fat margarine—remember, they added carbohydrates in place of the saturated fats in coconut oil. This group ended up with the worst combination of elevated total and LDL cholesterol, unchanged HDL and apoA-1, and the highest triglycerides of the bunch. The take-away? Although both unsaturated fats and coconut oil improved some measures of heart health, their effects differed. Perhaps there should be room in our diets for both types of fat? On the other hand, taking either kind of fat out of our diets and replacing them with carbohydrates might do our hearts the most harm.

Coconut and Weight

If the question of coconut and heart health has its complexities, the matter of coconut and weight control isn't exactly clear, either: For example, although coconut is very high in calories, the MCTs it contains seem to be associated with weight *loss*. In a randomized, double-blind study comparing equal doses of olive oil versus MCT oil (though not specifically coconut oil), fed to 31 subjects in muffins and cooking oil over the course of a 16-week weight-loss program, the group taking the MCT lost an average of 1.67 kg (3.7 pounds) *more* than the olive oil group, and their blood sugars, cholesterol, and blood pressure came out equal to those consuming the supposedly more heart-healthy olive oil.[48, 49] Unfortunately, the researchers did not track the subjects' other eating habits, so it is possible that other changes to their dietary factors could have been responsible for the coconut-positive results.

As for studies using actual coconut oil, recently an open-label (meaning unblinded) study by Malaysian researchers found that overweight men given a daily dose of virgin coconut oil lost an average of 2.86 cm (about an inch) from their waistlines in a four-week period.[50] As an open-label study, however, it lacked a control group to allow for direct comparisons. But the study did bring up the issue of the quality of coconut oil, which could be important: Like olive oil, coconut oil in its highest-quality form is known as virgin or extra-virgin coconut oil. As with so many unprocessed foods, the virgin form of coconut oil appears to be richer in nutrients and phytochemicals than the refined form. Unfortunately, much of the research to date has centred on coconut oils that may have been refined, or the type of coconut oil was not specified in the study. Only recently have researchers begun to clarify the difference between the two.

THE BOTTOM LINE

What we do know today about coconut suggests that, if you're looking for a food to lower your LDL cholesterol, you've probably come to the wrong place. Although coconut does seem to do some undesirable things to our lipid profiles—and it's worth noting that the best data we have to date suggests it increases *both* LDL and HDL—most of the population data we have suggests that it doesn't seem to be related to actual heart disease risk. As for the effects of coconut on weight loss, we simply don't have enough high-quality studies to say if the MCTs it contains are magical metabolizers or not, or what the optimal dose is. At the very least, coconut oil does not seem to cause weight gain, but it's still important to exchange coconut oil for other high-calorie foods (such as butter or plant oils) rather than take it as a supplement on top of your additional diet.

AGAVE NECTAR

Agave is everywhere. Touted in fitness magazines, in health blogs, and by celebrities, agave's big claim to fame is that it is a low-glycemic food, meaning it has a relatively small effect on blood sugar, especially compared with table sugar (sucrose). Since poorly controlled blood sugar is increasingly being linked to a variety of diseases and disorders, as well as chronic inflammation in the body, agave became the sweetener of choice for healthy gym-goers and foodies alike, including celebrity chef Giada De Laurentiis.[51]

AGAVE NECTAR: THE STORY

Agave nectar is a natural sweetener derived from the same plant as tequila. Also known as blue agave, or *Agave tequilana*, agave is from the same Asparagaceae family as asparagus. With spiky, succulent leaves, agave grows well at altitude and is primarily native to Mexico. Agave has a taste and texture similar to honey, so the two are often used interchangeably in recipes.

AGAVE NECTAR: THE NUTRITION

So how does agave stack up, nutritionally? Not as well as you might think: A tablespoon of agave provides about 60 calories' worth of energy, which is about 15 calories *more* than an equal serving of table sugar. Since agave is a more intense sweetener than sugar, however, the theory is you should be able to get away with using less of it. Its glycemic index (blood-sugar-raising effects, compared with pure glucose sugar) is, indeed, very low, with the GIs of various products ranging from 10 to 19 (anything under 55 is low; pure glucose sugar has a GI of 100).[52]

Now, here's the catch: Agave is very high in fructose (a recent analysis of 19 pure agave syrups found they contained an average of 84% fructose),[53] a type of sugar that doesn't convert to glucose and therefore doesn't raise blood sugar (the terms *blood sugar* and *blood glucose* are often used interchangeably). Fructose, however, which occurs naturally in fruit and honey (it also makes up about half of the sugar in table sugar and high-fructose corn syrup), happens to be on the nutrition naughty list these days, which means that agave, once the darling of sweeteners, has been kicked out of many kitchens, including that of health guru Dr. Andrew Weil.[54]

Why is fructose being given the cold shoulder? A body of research suggests that high-fructose diets can contribute to insulin resistance and high triglycerides, ultimately increasing our risk of developing heart disease and type 2 diabetes.[55] There are, however, a number of researchers who question the fructose-is-poison theory, at least significantly more so than other added sugars or refined carbohydrate foods.[56, 57, 58]

AGAVE NECTAR: THE SCIENCE

So what really happens when you feed someone agave? So far, the only studies on the effects of agave on metabolic health have been conducted in animals. In rats given free access to drinks sweetened with agave, high-fructose corn syrup (HFCS), or plain fructose every other day for 10 weeks (the researchers used an every-other-day design to mimic an average person's eating patterns), the rats taking the agave saw their triglycerides climb when compared with rats who spent the study drinking plain water.[59] The good news, however, is that their weight didn't change—in either direction. Interestingly, the agave group fared better than the HFCS or pure fructose groups, who ended up with higher cholesterol and triglycerides, as well as some elevated liver enzymes (an early sign of fatty liver), than their water-drinking counterparts. As far as animal studies go, this is far from a ringing endorsement for agave as a health food, but it also suggests that lumping agave together with HFCS and pure fructose might not be entirely fair.

Of course, food is complex, and any single food or ingredient contains numerous compounds, some of which can have positive and some of which can have negative impacts on our health. When it comes to agave, there is some muddiness: Despite the possible negative effects of the fructose in agave (which, to be fair, needs far more research, especially in humans), some of its fructose exists in a form known as a fructans, or long chain of fructose molecules. These fructans—the most well-known of which is inulin, a popular ingredient used to add fibre to cereals, granola bars, and even yogurt and cottage cheese—also occur in asparagus, leeks, onions, and chicory and are thought to have some health benefits for humans. In studies on rats, supplementing a regular diet with fructans from agave for five weeks prevented weight gain, increased appetite-suppressing hormones, reduced food intake, and reduced blood sugar and cholesterol levels versus rats fed a standard diet.[60] Interestingly, the amount of fructan also seems to increase as agave plants age,[61] so perhaps higher-quality agave from older plants could offer more health benefits than younger agave. Unfortunately, since studies such as these are looking at the fructans in isolation, it's hard to know just how comparable the results would be in whole foods, such as agave.

CONSEQUENCES OF CONSUMPTION

Like hemp, agave has some real potential to serve as an important energy source in a post-petroleum era. A special edition of the journal *GCB Biology* included a series of papers outlining the possible conversion of the remains of the agave plant into biofuels—after tequila production is complete, of course. Of concern is that the estimated cost of producing agave biofuel is much higher than that from corn or sugarcane, but it is hoped that, with greater efficiency, agave plants could eventually become a sustainable energy source.[63] Intriguingly, agave not only grows well in dry, nutrient-poor soil but also tolerates higher carbon dioxide levels in the air (it actually takes up substantial amounts of CO_2 at night and uses very limited amounts of water during the day). Since higher CO_2 levels are expected as the planet continues to warm, it is suggested that agave could be well suited to the conditions that climatologists predict will become more common as climate change takes hold.[64]

THE BOTTOM LINE

The agave story is, in some ways, a microcosm of our need to label foods as "good" or "bad," when neither side is actually true. Without at least a handful of well-controlled human trials, we simply don't know whether agave's lower GI could somehow be better for us than table sugar or if its high fructose content might do harm to our livers or triglycerides. For now, we have little more than theory. The bottom line, however, is that agave is still a form of sugar, and it's actually higher in calories than table sugar, so if you do decide to give this tricky little sweetener a try, you'd be well advised to do so sparingly.

WHEAT GRASS

Have you ever wondered why seemingly every juice and smoothie bar in North America has some kind of grass growing on the counter? That, my friends, is wheat grass, the same plant that would become wheat but is harvested before it turns into the golden grass we know so well. With the extraordinary nutrition claims that surround it, wheat grass can be a lightning rod for both health enthusiasts and skeptics alike. So what do we know about this grass that is said to be an energy-boosting cure-all? At the very least, it has a unique, and intriguing, history.

WHEAT GRASS: THE STORY

The popularity of wheat grass (*Triticum aestivum*) stems from the work of Charles F. Schnabel, an agricultural chemist from Missouri whose early work focused on improving the quality of animal feeds. In the 1920s, Schnabel took interest in the health properties of young shoots from cereal grasses, including barley and rye but most especially wheat. According to Schnabel's research, wheat grass that is harvested before jointing, the stage when the newly formed seed starts to migrate up the shoot, is higher in nutrients than the more mature version of itself, and it is also nutritionally superior to other common vegetables. After jointing, Schnabel argued, the nutritional value of the grass declines as the nutrients are shunted toward the newly forming seeds; for example, he found that the protein content of the grass declined from 40% to 30% after jointing. As such, Schnabel believed that early cereal grasses could make a suitable addition to the diet, either fresh or as a supplement, of humans and animals. Schnabel's enthusiasm for wheat grass was so great that he applied for, and was granted, a patent for processing the grass shoots in 1934.[65]

Schnabel's efforts eventually led him to develop Cerophyl, one of the earliest-known multivitamin supplements. Derived from dried wheat grass, Cerophyl was a powdered supplement taken in pill form and reportedly rich in vitamins A, B, E, and K.[66] Although Cerophyl experienced tremendous popularity in the 1940s, it had one big downside: The sheer volume of the freeze-dried powdered wheat grass meant the recommended dose was a cumbersome 20 capsules per day. Eventually, the development of synthetic vitamin supplements, taken only once daily, signalled Cerophyl's demise in the wider market.

Nonetheless, wheat grass persisted, and in the 1970s it enjoyed a resurgence in the burgeoning health food industry. A small company, known as PINES International, reintroduced dehydrated wheat grass, grown in the nutrient-rich postglacial soil of Kansas, to the mass market; among its early clients was a group of health food stores that eventually merged to become Whole Foods. In 2012, PINES obtained the Cerophyl trademark and, in a twist of fate, ended up purchasing Schnabel's old Cerophyl production facility.[67]

Although PINES still produces wheat grass supplements grown

in northeastern Kansas, more recently, fresh wheat grass has become available to consumers, grown indoors in trays. Although field-grown wheat grass grows slowly over the winter months, trayed wheat grass is harvested in about 10 days, a point of criticism among some wheat grass aficionados, who argue that dark green, field-grown wheat grass is far more nutrient dense than the pale green grass you'll find growing indoors in a tray.

WHEAT GRASS: THE NUTRITION

Although the 1930s and '40s featured an abundance of research on wheat grass (or wheat juice, as it was often called), to date, wheat grass is not included in the USDA National Nutrient Database or the Canadian Nutrient File. As a result, consumers are left to piece together information on wheat grass from wheat grass retailers, by gathering nuggets of data from old research papers (many of which were published before all the known vitamins had been identified), or through books published on the subject. Notably, much of what we know about wheat grass comes from grass grown in nutrient-rich fields; it is difficult to say how it stacks up when grown in a tray, but PINES claims tray-grown wheat grass is significantly lower in vitamin A, folic acid, iron, calcium, and potassium.[68]

According to PINES, 1 teaspoon of dried wheat grass (3.5 grams, or seven tablets) provides about 1 gram of protein, 8% of your vitamin A, 10% of your vitamin C, and 5% of your folic acid needs for the day, along with 137 mg of potassium.[69] It is also said to be rich in vitamin K and chlorophyll, the green pigment that acts as the site of photosynthesis in plants. More recent analysis has identified the presence of numerous active plant compounds, including flavonoids, triterpenoids, quinols, alkaloids, and cholesterol-lowering sterols, as well as less-desirable nutrient-binding compounds such as saponins and tannins.[70] Unfortunately, the effects of these phytochemicals present in wheat grass have yet to be established. Interestingly, unlike mature wheat, wheat grass is said to be gluten free.

WHEAT GRASS: THE SCIENCE

The science of wheat grass can largely be categorized in two groups: the early studies, conducted by a group of agricultural scientists on a variety of animals in the 1930s and '40s, and more recent research, which is relatively limited and covers a fairly small number of health conditions.

The early research centred on the observation of many farmers that their animals fared best when eating fresh spring grass versus dried winter rations. Specifically, the milk produced by cows was the most nutritious in the summer months, when they had recent access to young, unjointed wheat grass in pastures, versus the winter, when the grass they ate had passed the point of jointing and came in the form of dried mature hay. In 1936, a group of researchers, including C.A. Elvehjem, found that supplementing 3 ml of spring grass juice to rats otherwise fed winter milk increased their growth to more than 4 grams per day, a rate comparable to the rats' growth on summer milk.[71] In follow-up studies, Elvehjem and colleagues, including George C. Kohler, tried to isolate what made wheat juice so effective at stimulating growth.[72] After eliminating various B vitamins, as well as vitamins A, D, and C (vitamins E and K had not yet been identified), choline, and other "factors" known at the time, the researchers ran out of options. It seems they simply couldn't identify what, exactly, made the grass juice so special.

The conundrum persisted. In 1939, the *Journal of the American Medical Association* reviewed E.Y. McCallum's *The Newer Knowledge of Nutrition*, a book that included references to as-yet unexplained factors in growth, including the "grass juice factor."[73] And while other elements, such as vitamin K, have since been identified and may play some role in the benefits obtained from wheat grass, no one has been able to fully explain just how grass harvested before jointing helped the animals grow and thrive better than wheat eaten after jointing.

Although the early days of research on wheat grass were certainly interesting, only a handful of studies have examined its effects in humans since then. In fact, using the search terms "wheat grass" or "wheat juice" reveals only six clinical trials in PubMed, one of the primary search engines for medical research. Of the six trials, only one is a randomized, double-blind, placebo-controlled trial, the highest quality of clinical research. In this study, the effect of daily supplementation with 100 ml of wheat grass juice was examined versus placebo on 23 patients with ulcerative colitis.[74] After a month of supplementation, those taking the wheat grass experienced a significant reduction in overall disease activity index as well as the severity of rectal bleeding. Despite a long history of purported bowel health benefits, this remains the only controlled trial to assess the benefits of wheat grass on the human digestive system.

Otherwise, a number of studies have examined the effects of wheat grass juice on iron status, especially in individuals with thalassemia, a genetically transferred form of anemia that may require transfusions. A pilot study conducted in India found that, among 16 patients with thalassemia major who consumed approximately 100 ml of wheat grass juice daily, eight saw their needs for blood transfusion reduced by at least one-quarter, and three patients saw their need decline by more than 40%.[75] Unfortunately, the study was not well controlled in a variety of ways (for example, the subjects grew their own wheat grass rather than receiving a standardized supplement) and had a low level of compliance, which was attributed to the effort required to grow, harvest, and extract the juice.

Aside from the small number of human studies, some studies on animals suggest wheat grass could have cholesterol-lowering effects. Two studies on rats, for example, conducted by the same research group, demonstrated a dose-dependent effect of wheat grass on total cholesterol, LDL cholesterol, and triglycerides, with a large dose (equal to about 3 cups of wheat grass a day) resulting in a cholesterol-lowering effect on par with simvastatin, or Zocor.[76, 77] A similar study demonstrated both lipid-lowering and antioxidant effects of wheat grass on rabbits.[78]

Finally, there is also some evidence that wheat grass juice may reduce some side effects of chemotherapy. In a pilot study on 60 patients receiving chemotherapy for breast cancer, daily supplementation with 60 ml (about 2 ounces) of wheat grass during the first three cycles of chemotherapy reduced the need for additional costly and side-effect-provoking therapies, yet itself without decreasing the effectiveness of the chemotherapy.[79] Since this is a pilot study, however, high-quality placebo-controlled trials, conducted with various types of cancer, are necessary to confirm this initial finding.

THE BOTTOM LINE

Wheat grass is a rare superfood that garnered more interest from the scientific community some 70-plus years ago than it does now. No doubt, the early research is intriguing: What, exactly, was the cause of that impressive growth observed by animals fed young (unjointed) wheat grass? And could those seemingly health-promoting effects translate into benefits for humans? Unfortunately, we still have more questions than answers. As a result, it's not entirely surprising that wheat grass is so polarizing; although some remain understandably skeptical due to the dearth of information, others see wheat grass as having vast, untapped potential to improve human health.

3

SMEAR CAMPAIGN

SUPERFOODS WITH AN UNFAIRLY BAD RAP

Beef? Potatoes? Cheese? If the thought of adding these foods to your superfood list makes you feel about as healthy as a couple of days of chain smoking, then this next chapter might leave you feeling a bit woozy. But if you at least let yourself sink into the debate a little, you might be surprised at how you feel when you come out on the other side. Remember, there was once a time when we thought that almost any fat was bad for us, leaving so many of us feeling queasy or decadent at the thought of using real oil for salad dressing or cooking. As with many issues in nutrition, the story of these controversial superfoods is mired in conflicting data, and although there are rarely black-and-white answers, there is a case to be made that these foods deserve better than their current reputation suggests.

BEEF

Putting beef on a superfood list is a surefire way to ruffle some feathers. Long viewed as some kind of nutritional pornography—a naughty pleasure that you enjoy when your wife's not around—beef has been on the downswing in terms of public image for decades. Yet somehow, when you look at its nutrition profile, the idea that beef might be so darn bad for you can seem a little hard to swallow.

BEEF: THE NUTRITION

Since each cut of beef's marbling (fat content) is distinct, its nutrition content will vary. Some cuts, such as round and eye of round, are very lean, which means they are not only low in total fat, they are also low in saturated fat, the type of fat that has long been said to be harmful to our hearts. Other cuts, especially those from the rib (think rib-eye and prime rib), are heavily marbled and as such are higher in fat, saturated fat, and, by extension, calories (a gram of fat provides more than double the 4 calories per gram provided by a gram of protein or carbohydrate, so even modest variations in fat content of a food can have a significant effect on its calorie content). For simplicity's sake, then, let's use the sirloin, a middle-of-the-road cut, to take a closer look at beef's nutritional value.

A 100-gram (3.5 ounce) serving of cooked sirloin steak, which is about the size of the palm of your hand, provides 193 calories' worth of energy, along with 26 grams of protein. Beef is an excellent source of niacin (vitamin B_3) and vitamin B_6, providing 39% and 27%, respectively, of your daily needs for each. Like many animal foods, beef is also an excellent source of vitamin B_{12}, providing about a quarter of your daily needs (27%) per serving. Although it's well known that beef is rich in iron, the 10% of your daily requirements that it provides might seem a little ho-hum. Compared with plant-based iron sources, however, beef and other animal foods contain a type of iron known as heme iron, which is absorbed about three times better than the plant form of iron, known as non-heme iron. In other words, deriving 10% of your needs from beef is about the same as receiving 30% of your requirements from a plant food, which is a very rare find. Beef is also particularly rich in zinc (a third of your needs for a day), as well as the antioxidant selenium (43%).

BEEF: THE SCIENCE

There are a handful of reasons why beef and, more broadly, red meat have been given the nutritional heave-ho. Let's take a look at each.

Beef and Heart Disease

Yes, it's true: Beef does contain saturated fat, and the fattier the cut of beef, the higher the number goes. And yes, it's also true that, to this day, public health recommendations encourage us to reduce our intake of saturated fat, limiting it to less than 20 grams, or about 10% of our total calories, per day, and it's widely accepted that dietitians such as me should educate our clients to reduce their intake of saturated fats to cut their risk of heart disease. Unfortunately, what once seemed like a straightforward strategy to help people control their cholesterol now seems muddier, leaving many of us caught between following the recommendations and rapidly evolving research.

Before we even get to the evidence on saturated fat, let's first consider that in recent years we have seen a number of studies suggesting that higher-protein, lower-carbohydrate diets—which beef can figure into quite nicely—are at least equal to low-fat diets for weight loss, and in some cases, the low-carbohydrate diets produced better results related to heart health.[1, 2, 3] On top of that, in 2006 a fascinating study, published in the *American Journal of Clinical Nutrition*, suggested that although carbohydrates don't necessarily affect the total amount of

LDL cholesterol they do cause an increase in small, dense LDL—that fraction of LDL that is considered the most harmful.[4] Two years later, a landmark study known as the OmniHeart Trial found that when subjects increased their intake of protein in exchange for either carbohydrate or unsaturated fat (yes, the "good" fat), their apoB levels—remember, that's a marker of the small, dense LDL—dropped, as did their levels of another compound associated with some of the nastiest fats in our bloodstreams, known as apolipoprotein C-III (apoC-III).[5]

Since we already knew that eating a diet higher in carbohydrates could trigger a jump in triglycerides, another fat associated with heart disease risk, we now had increasingly convincing evidence that the low-fat, high-carbohydrate way of thinking (think of all the packages of sugary candy that proudly declare themselves as "low fat" or "fat free") might have done both our hearts and our waistlines more harm than good.

Even though some health care professionals and researchers started to question the validity of the low-fat way of thinking, it was still widely accepted that the only "good" fat was unsaturated, such as that found in avocados, olive oil, nuts, and seeds. More recently, however, several leading researchers suggested that saturated fat isn't harmful to us after all.[6, 7, 8] At its core, the issue seems to be about what we do when we cut saturated fats: If we take them out and use polyunsaturated fats in exchange, our heart health profile tends to improve. When we replace saturated fats with carbohydrates, however, our hearts don't win: Instead, our triglycerides go up, our HDL ("good" cholesterol) goes down, and, as mentioned, we produce more small, dense LDL.[9, 10]

As for the red meat issue in particular, despite years of research suggesting that red meat is linked with heart disease, a trio of researchers from Harvard found that the way red meat is processed could play an important role in its effect on health.[11] After analyzing the 20 best-designed studies they could find, the researchers found that, instead of lumping all red meat together (as had been done in previous studies), processed red meat was associated with a 42% higher risk of heart disease and a 19% higher risk of diabetes per 50 grams consumed per day, but unprocessed red meat was *not* associated with heart disease, stroke, or diabetes risk. Since then, a cohort study found that while processed meat was associated with diabetes risk in American Indians, unprocessed meat was not.[12]

But let's take the discussion one step farther. Let's just assume for a moment that saturated fat is, actually, bad for us and that red meat, by extension, does our hearts some harm. Then there is the issue of how the meat we eat is raised. Since Michael Pollan's *The Omnivore's Dilemma*[13] introduced so many of us to the impact of feedlot animals on our food supply, there has been an increasing awareness of the importance of an animal's diet not only for the animal's health and well-being, but also for the humans who consume it. Specifically, research has demonstrated that beef from grass-fed (i.e., pasture-raised) cows tends to be lower in saturated fat, be richer in omega-3 fatty acids, and contain more conjugated linoleic acid (CLA)—a compound that is naturally produced by ruminant animals and that may be protective against heart disease and certain cancers—than beef from traditional feedlots.[14] Yet, because very few people eat grass-fed beef, and many of those who do likely began doing so only recently, the big population studies we have are mostly based on beef and red meat that have been industrially produced, with the less-desirable fat profile that goes along with it.

So let's turn this around and put it another way: In this day and age, when saturated fat from red meat means eating a hamburger on a white bun with fries and pop after a tough day of sitting around at the office, it's easy to see why beef can look so ugly. On the other hand, eating a moderate portion of grass-fed beef sliced over a spinach salad a few times per week could have a completely different effect on our health. Of course, science rarely shifts overnight, so to this day, many well-regarded researchers still staunchly believe we need to cut our intake of saturated fat to reduce our risk of heart disease, but there are many who feel less confident in these recommendations than even a couple of years ago.

Beef and Cancer Risk

Unfortunately, the controversy around beef doesn't end with heart disease: There is also concern that red meat raises cancer risk. The concern stems from two possible triggers: the heme iron in beef interacting with high heat, such as the flames on a barbecue, to produce carcinogens, as well as the interaction of the nitrates added to cured and processed meats, which is also thought to produce cancer-causing compounds. Taken together, a major systematic review by the World Cancer Research Fund and the American Institute for Cancer Research declared there was "convincing" evidence that red meat is associated with colorectal cancer risk.[15] Despite the strength of these findings, however, a few questions still remain. First, the research used for these meta-analyses is largely based on population studies, which rely on having subjects fill out questionnaires about what they eat, sometimes only once (at the start of the study) or on a semi-regular basis (e.g., every couple of years). The researchers then try to correlate the results with health or disease outcomes. Ideally, the questionnaires—which are used because they are less costly and easier to administer than other methods of assessing diet, such as in-person interviews—are tested against other, more reliable dietary assessment tools to make sure their results are valid. Even when the questionnaires are validated, however, their use spurs endless debate in the scientific community; not everyone is convinced that they give us enough reliable information to allow us to make population health recommendations.

Aside from the use of questionnaires, another concern with many population studies is that they often lump all forms of red meat, be it processed or unprocessed, into one big pile. That makes it awfully difficult to untangle the effects of bologna versus beef tenderloin, especially when cured meats contain nitrates that might have a carcinogenic effect (interestingly, however, the nitrates we get from fruits and vegetables—which make up the vast majority of our nitrate intake—don't seem to do us any harm). Also notable is the fact that cooking red meats with marinades, herbs, and spices seems to reduce the production of carcinogens, but these sorts of details are rarely captured in population studies. All of this is to say that what we do with our meat, not to mention how we raise it, might have a big effect on how it works in our bodies. This also takes us back to the issue of other health behaviours that come along with red meat intake; we know, for example, that vegetarians tend to be healthier than meat eaters, but they also tend to eat better diets overall and exercise more, and they are less likely to smoke. Likewise, if red meat eaters just don't treat themselves very well, then a higher risk of cancer is a possible corollary—but it might not be because of the meat.

Beef and Your Muscles

Although the questions about beef and cancer are bewitching, some research about beef is fairly black and white: As with other meats, poultry, and fish, beef has real potential benefit when it comes to building and maintaining muscle and to preventing what is known as sarcopenia, or age-related muscle loss. This all relates back to how our bodies build muscle and how protein works to support the process.

At any moment in time, our bodies are constantly building up or breaking down the all-important muscle tissue that not only helps keep us strong but also maintains our balance, helps us age well, and speeds our metabolism. When we build up more muscle protein than we break down, we can expect to hang onto, or even build, new muscle over a period of time. On the other hand, when we break down more muscle protein than we are building, we can start to lose muscle. Over short periods of time—a few hours or even a few days—the difference between building up (anabolism) and breaking down (catabolism) muscle is pretty slight (though high-level athletes generally want to spend as little time as possible in the catabolic, or breakdown, state). When multiplied over weeks, months, and years, however, the net effect of that muscle breakdown, or catabolism, can lead to a real, noticeable loss of muscle—think of the effects of wearing a cast on an arm or a leg as an example. For this reason, challenging our bodies to build, or at least maintain, muscle rather than break it down is of great importance, whether it's for dieters (who tend to lose muscle while restricting their eating), active individuals (the more activity you do, the faster the buildup and breakdown rates become), or anyone who happens to be getting older—which, I'm pretty sure, is all of us. There are two ways to accomplish this: through diet, particularly by eating foods containing protein, and through exercise, especially resistance or strength training. The best bet, of course, is to do both.

It is exactly the first part of that equation—how much protein we can use at one time to put us at the positive end of building up muscle, also known as muscle protein synthesis (MPS)—that University of

Texas researchers, including Drs. Robert R. Wolfe and Douglas Paddon-Jones, have been trying to answer. In an already-classic study examining protein intake at a single meal, they compared the effects of eating 113 grams (about 4 ounces) of lean beef, providing 30 grams of protein, versus a larger serving (340 grams of meat, or about a 12 ounce steak), providing about 90 grams of protein, on rates of MPS.[16] In effect, they wanted to find out just how much protein a person could eat in one sitting to max out their ability to build muscle. Their finding was intriguing: Eating 90 grams of protein (the amount in the 12 ounce steak) had a clear benefit on MPS, but its effect was no greater than that received from eating just 30 grams of protein (the amount in the palm-sized serving of beef). Perhaps even more significant were results suggesting that eating less than 20 grams of protein per meal can blunt muscle protein synthesis (allowing your body's protein balance to tip into the negative, or breakdown, mode). This negative effect of eating too little protein seems to be especially pronounced in older adults, who are prone to what is known as sarcopenia, or age-related muscle loss.[17] In other words, although a younger person can get away with missing out on protein at mealtime with only limited effects on muscle, in an older adult, eating protein at regular intervals seems to be particularly crucial to keep muscles from breaking down. As a result of our new understanding of protein's role in successful aging, there is a growing movement to re-evaluate our nutrient recommendations for older adults to include a higher dietary reference intake for protein.[18]

Now, before you go off and start celebrating by grilling a side of beef for dinner, remember this research suggests that you max out your benefit by eating about 20 to 30 grams of protein—once again, that's about a palm-sized serving of meat—per meal. By comparison, that 12-ounce porterhouse may offer no more benefit, at least in terms of muscle protein synthesis, than a more modest filet, but it sure will cost both you and the environment a whole lot more. Translation? Although some groups, such as the elderly, might do well to push their protein intake a bit more, the rest of us would do well to balance our protein throughout the day while still exercising that all-important portion control.

THE BOTTOM LINE

It's hard not to believe our ancestors had a pretty good idea of what our bodies need to survive and thrive. Red meat has been a part of the human diet since time immemorial, so it does seem a little odd that it is such a hazard to our health. It's possible that beef's benefits have been drowned out by the feed we give our cows or by confusion over the role that the lousy carbohydrates that we eat with our beef play in our health. Put another way: What if the issue isn't the hamburger but the bun? What we once thought was true needs some rethinking.

CHEESE

Cheese as a superfood? That sounds about as reasonable as having potato chips or gummy bears on the list. Yet somehow, cheese seems to be making a small comeback as more and more people tune in to some of its underappreciated yet distinct properties that could have important benefits for our health.

CHEESE: THE STORY

Cheese-making is as old as recorded history or perhaps even older. It's thought that humans stumbled across cheese-making when they used the stomachs of animals, such as sheep, to transport milk (the world's first biodegradable shopping bag?). It's in the stomach of sheep, cows, and other animals that the enzyme rennet exists, which, we now understand, helps curdled milk (which naturally separates into curds and whey protein) coagulate into the gel that is young, unripened cheese. Our ancestors learned quickly that cheese had benefits that extended beyond milk, as it was more portable and had a longer shelf life than milk itself. By the time of the Roman Empire, cheese-making was well established in Europe, the Middle East, and parts of South Asia, with a reach extending as far east as Tibet.

The process of cheese-making requires the use of not only soured milk and rennet but also bacteria, which, through the aging process, give cheese its distinct flavours. The bacteria in cheese convert the natural milk sugar, lactose, into lactic acid, which means that cheese, especially aged hard cheeses, such as old cheddar, is less likely to trigger the bloating and stomach pain that are usually associated with lactose intolerance.

CHEESE: THE NUTRITION

When it comes to cheese, less is more. Although we might measure portions of milk, fruit, and vegetables in cups, the high calorie content of cheese means that serving sizes are usually just 30 grams (about an ounce) while Canada's Food Guide uses a reference serving size of 50 grams, an amount that will provide you with about the same amount of calcium as a cup of milk or 3/4 cup of yogurt. For a 50-gram serving size, then, you can expect 201 calories and 17 grams of fat, of which almost 11 grams are the much-maligned saturated fats, along with 13 grams of protein. The top vitamins and minerals in cheese are calcium (357 mg, or 36% of your daily needs), vitamin A, vitamin B$_2$, zinc, and selenium (11% of each). Since cheese is salted, it also tends to be fairly high in sodium, with about 300 mg (about 1/8 of your daily limit) per 50-gram serving.

CHEESE: THE SCIENCE

As a result of health recommendations to reduce our intake of saturated fat, which naturally occurs in dairy products, we've subsisted off of 0% yogurt (the percent reflects the percentage of calories from fat), skim milk (my Dutch friend calls this grey water), and low-fat cheese, the latter of which provides the culinary delights of chewing on a flat tire. More recently, however, researchers have been re-examining the data we have on dairy products, and the findings could turn nutrition upside down: If you look carefully at the available evidence, it is now being argued that there is actually no link between consuming full-fat dairy and the risk of heart disease.[19, 20, 21] In fact, the opposite might be true: Higher-fat dairy (and in some cases, cheese specifically) could, seemingly paradoxically, be associated with a *lower* risk of cardiovascular disease.[22, 23, 24]

If it turns out these findings are, in fact, true, it begs the question, how could we have been so wrong? A big part of the problem could be that cheese and full-fat dairy foods tend to be associated with a lower-quality diet, at least in the United States. When researchers looked at dietary patterns in the U.S. population, they found that full-fat dairy is more commonly consumed by people who are at a higher risk of heart disease and diabetes. Fair enough, but as it turns out, the same people who eat full-fat dairy in the United States are also more likely to smoke, be overweight, be inactive, and eat a lower-quality diet. If you go to Europe, on the other hand, eating full-fat dairy is a part of life and is actually associated with a higher-quality diet and healthier lifestyle.

In other words, it might not be the cheese that's the problem but rather the company it tends to keep. In the United States, that is more likely to be burgers on white buns, pop, and cigarettes; in Europe, it is greens, fruit, and red wine. The difference, healthwise, between these two diets is drastic.

Although there are some basic nutrients in cheese that are important for health, such as protein, calcium, and vitamin A, cheese also has an underappreciated but perhaps even more important ingredient that could play a vital role in human health, and that is bacteria. Cheese, like yogurt, is a fermented food product, which means bacteria are involved in its conversion from liquid milk to solid food. Unlike yogurt, however, the benefit from eating cheese is derived not from the live bacteria but rather from the by-products the bacteria produce during the aging process, most specifically vitamin K_2, or more technically, menaquinone.

Vitamin K_2 is a family of compounds of various sizes, ranging from MK_1 (MK refers to menaquinone) to MK_{14}. We'll get into vitamin K_1 in the section on kale, but for now, let's keep it to this: Vitamin K_1, known as phylloquinone, long known as a vital factor for blood clotting, is also being lauded for its potential anti-inflammatory and insulin-modulating effects. Vitamin K_2, however, is generating its own share of attention, especially for its potential role in heart health. The turning point for vitamin K_2 might have been in 2004, when Dutch researchers published a study suggesting that individuals with the highest intake of vitamin K_2 had a 57% lower risk of dying of heart disease, and a 26% lower risk of dying from any cause, than those with the lowest intake.[25] The high-vitamin-K_2 group were also much less likely to have calcified arteries (arteries made rigid by the buildup of calcium) than groups with the lowest levels. Interestingly, vitamin K_1, which is found mostly in green, leafy vegetables, was not associated with any of these benefits. A few years later, the same research team proposed what is known as a dose–response effect for vitamin K_2 and heart health, meaning that as K_2 intake increases, heart disease risk drops in a linear fashion (more precisely, for every 10 micrograms per day of vitamin K_2 consumed, the odds of developing heart disease dropped by about 9%).[26]

Why could vitamin K_2 be so important for our hearts? The answer could lie with calcium. As mentioned, too much calcium in our arteries could leave us more prone to heart attacks, a fact that is a source of much irritation for women who are repeatedly told they need more calcium, only to see studies come out suggesting that too much calcium from supplements might actually increase the risk for heart attacks. According to the emerging theory, calcium, in a way, needs to be "told" where to go. That's where vitamin K_2 comes in: Its job is to direct calcium to the right places, namely to our bones, and not to the wrong places, namely our arteries. It does this by changing the way key proteins in our bones and our hearts work, through a process known as carboxylation. In our hearts, vitamin K_2 carboxylates a key protein known as MGP (short for matrix Gla-protein—good news: there is no test on this), which prevents calcium from being laid down in our arteries, while in our bones, vitamin K_2 carboxylates a protein known as calcitonin, which then activates bone-building cells known as osteoblasts. Sure enough, a systematic review and meta-analysis of seven studies found that vitamin K_2 supplementation helped prevent bone loss and reduced risk of fracture.[27] The effect of vitamin K_2 might also explain why we see some inconsistencies in the vitamin D research: Vitamin D's job is to help our bodies absorb calcium, but if we don't have enough vitamin K_2, then that calcium might not know where to go. It might not be enough to have one without the other.

But the intrigue doesn't end there: There is also evidence that vitamin K_2 could play a role in cancer prevention. U.S. researchers, for example, have made the connection between vitamin K_2 and prostate cancer,[28] while there is considerable research suggesting that dairy foods, and specifically high-fat ones, might be protective against colorectal cancer.[29]

So, where do you get vitamin K_2? Why, cheese, of course.[30] Before you get too excited, however, the amount of vitamin K_2 in cheese is far less than that found in the fermented Japanese soybean product natto (no doubt worthy of its own superfood section—save that for the next book), though they exist as different forms of vitamin K_2 (natto typically provides MK_7, while cheese provides MK_8 and MK_9), the implications for which are not yet entirely clear.[31] Other smaller vitamin K_2 sources include eggs (in the yolk), liver, beef, and chicken, and we also convert a small amount of vitamin K_1 to K_2 in our digestive tracts.

So, which cheeses should we eat? Again, we have much to learn. So far, it is suggested that aged and ripened cheeses, such as aged cheddar, Brie, and Gouda, provide the most vitamin K_2. Young cheese, such as ricotta and mozzarella, may provide very little, if any. Processed cheese may contain very small amounts of vitamin K_2,[32] which might mean that if the cheese you eat comes from cheese slices, cheese spreads, pizza, nachos, or deep-fried cheese sticks, you might not be getting much vitamin K_2 at all. These findings could help (finally) explain the French paradox, namely that the French, who routinely eat full-fat dairy foods and drink wine, tend to have a relatively low heart disease risk: They might be getting some of the benefit by enjoying quality cheeses with their meals.

THE BOTTOM LINE

As I said at the start of this book, my fear in labelling foods "super-foods" is that we will unfairly elevate one food above another. In this case, I hope you will heed my words and not chase your next meal with a half-pound of double-cream Brie. Much of the evidence we have to date is built on correlations and associations rather than on the best kind of evidence that comes from randomized, controlled trials. It's simply too early to give clear guidelines, and it's also worth noting that, in the Dutch study mentioned earlier, those with the highest intake of vitamin K$_2$ also had a *higher* body weight. Yes, good-quality cheese might be delicious and, as it turns out, more nutritious than we once thought, but it is still calorie dense, meaning that if you want to add it to your diet, you need to do it in place of something else.

COCOA AND DARK CHOCOLATE

Is there really any controversy to cocoa? You might think not, but you'll still hear rumblings from the medical establishment that giving a nod to cocoa could lead to us consuming too many calories and too much supposedly artery-clogging saturated fat. Well established in many circles as a top-notch choice, both for its mineral content and for its phytochemicals (active plant compounds) that are associated with better health and a reduced risk of disease, cocoa has become something of a darling in recent years. But a few issues obscure the cocoa picture, particularly the way it is usually delivered: namely, as chocolate. So, is it fair to call cocoa a superfood? That depends on how you look at it.

COCOA: THE STORY

Cocoa, and ultimately chocolate, is derived from the cacao plant that is part of the *Theobroma* family. With a long history of use that dates back to 1600 B.C., cocoa was often made into beverages by the Aztecs, including a fermented liquid cocoa that they dubbed *chocolatl*. The Incas considered cocoa to be a drink of the gods, which helps explain how the cocoa plant, or *Theobroma cacao*—*theo* meaning god and *broma* meaning drink—got its name.[33] European explorers ultimately took interest in the bitter cocoa beverage, bringing it back to their native land, where the roots of commercial chocolate production took hold.

Of course, cocoa powder itself has many uses, including chocolate, but also hot cocoa, which can easily be made on the stove, using nothing more than cocoa powder, milk, a bit of sugar, and vanilla or other flavourings. Cocoa can also be used in uncommon pairings, especially in chili and other savoury dishes native to Central and South America.

COCOA: THE NUTRITION

A tablespoon of dry, unsweetened cocoa powder provides just 12 calories' worth of energy, along with a hint of fat (0.7 gram total, of which 0.4 gram is saturated) and a surprisingly decent 1.7 grams of fibre. If you're looking for vitamins in cocoa, you've come to the wrong place, but its mineral content isn't bad for the small portion, at 4% of your daily iron, 7% of your magnesium, and 10% of your copper. You'll also pick up about 12 mg of caffeine, which is about one-quarter of the amount in a cup of tea.

If, however, you decide to down a full ounce of plain cocoa (remember that cocoa is, shall we say, rather less sweet than chocolate), which is about half the weight of a typical chocolate bar, the nutritional value would leapfrog into the upper echelons, with 9 grams of fibre, 5 grams of protein, 22% of your daily iron, 35% of your magnesium, 427 mg (12%) of your potassium, 13% of your zinc, and more than half of your daily copper needs packed into just 64 calories, or about the same number as you'd get from a small orange.

Fine, that's a nice story, but let's be honest: Most of us are here to find out what happens when we get to the good stuff. If you switch from pure cocoa to a 1-ounce serving of dark chocolate made from 70% to 85% cocoa solids, you're now on the hook for 168 calories and 12 grams of fat, of which 7 are saturated, along with 7 grams (just under 2 teaspoons) of sugar. The fibre content is still reasonable at 3 grams, along with 2 grams of protein. Although the vitamin content is, once again, negligible, an ounce of dark chocolate is still a good source of the minerals iron (19%), magnesium (16%), and copper (25%) and provides 200 mg of potassium, or about half the amount in a banana. The caffeine content comes in at 22 mg, less than half the amount in a cup of tea.

But what if the semi-bitter taste of dark chocolate, especially at the high end of the range, simply isn't your thing? Choosing milk chocolate not only means adding more sugar (about 13 grams for an ounce of chocolate with about 50% cocoa solids—remember, a typical chocolate bar is about twice that size), but you'll also lose one-third to half of the top minerals, including iron, magnesium, and copper. In other words, for chocolate to be considered a superfood, it really has to be dark.

COCOA: THE SCIENCE

In traditional medicine, cocoa has been used to prevent and treat a variety of diseases and illnesses, including anemia (presumably because of its iron content), fatigue (perhaps due, at least in part, to its caffeine content), gout, and even tuberculosis.[34] To date, however, these traditional uses have not been validated in well-designed human research. The best evidence we have centres instead around blood pressure and cardiovascular disease, both of which seem to be impacted by diets that contain cocoa.

Cocoa and Blood Pressure

Some of our interest in the effects of cocoa on blood pressure stems from research on the Kuna Indians, who live on the San Blas archipelago off the shores of Panama. Unlike so many cultures, the Kuna do not seem to experience age-related blood pressure changes or declines in kidney function, and their death rate from cardiovascular events (about 9 age-adjusted deaths per 100,000 people) is drastically lower than that of mainlanders (83/100,000). Although it might be assumed that the Kuna are simply genetically resistant to blood pressure changes and cardiovascular disease, their metabolic advantages disappear once they migrate to the mainland.[35] So, what makes the Kuna so special? There are many possibilities, including their traditional plant-based diet, but the Kuna are particularly noted for consuming enormous amounts of cocoa.[36]

Now, that's all well and good, but hopefully by now you've picked up on a pattern, namely that the research on the Kuna speaks only to correlation, not causation. To establish that cocoa actually causes a change in blood pressure, we need well-designed randomized, controlled trials. In this case, we are in luck: A 2012 *Cochrane Review* found that 20 studies, involving 856 mainly healthy subjects, were good enough to be included in their systematic review (it's unusual to see that many well-designed studies related to a single food). When the data from these studies was combined, the researchers found that daily consumption of cocoa-rich products had a small effect on blood pressure, roughly amounting to a drop of 2 or 3 points (mm Hg, or mercury) in both systolic and diastolic blood pressure. For reasons that are not entirely clear, the effect seems to be strongest in shorter-term studies (usually two weeks or less).[37] Although that number isn't necessarily eye-popping (healthy blood pressure is under 120/80; high blood pressure, or hypertension, is diagnosed after blood pressure consistently exceeds 140/90), it at least suggests that cocoa-rich foods aren't harmful to blood pressure, and the effects are on par with several other interventions to lower blood pressure. In other words, eating cocoa on its own probably won't keep you from developing high blood pressure, but combined with other healthy habits, such as eating more fruits and vegetables, losing weight, and exercising, cocoa could fit into a healthy diet pattern that would support a healthy heart.

Cocoa and Other CVD Risk Factors

Beyond high blood pressure, there is also some evidence that cocoa could be protective against cardiovascular disease in general. In a study of 470 elderly men free from chronic disease, those with the highest intake of cocoa had a 47% lower risk of all-cause mortality than those who consumed the least.[38] As for clinical trials, a meta-analysis (a compilation and re-analysis of data from previous studies) of 42 studies, published in the *American Journal of Clinical Nutrition*, found that daily consumption of cocoa, chocolate, or flavan-3-ols (the active compounds in cocoa) reduced insulin resistance and improved something known as flow-mediated dilation, a measure of the capacity of the arteries to dilate and allow blood flow throughout the body, when compared with consuming no cocoa at all.[39] The authors also noted a trend toward a drop in LDL ("bad") cholesterol and a similar increase in HDL cholesterol, but the effects weren't big enough to be considered statistically significant. A smaller meta-analysis, involving

10 trials with 320 participants ranging from 2 to 12 weeks, did find that cocoa products and dark chocolate were associated with a small but significant drop in LDL (averaging about 0.15 mmol/L) and total cholesterol, but the study did not see an effect on HDL cholesterol.[40] Taken together, this data suggests that, as with blood pressure, the effect that cocoa or chocolate has on cholesterol is probably small, but it seems to have neutral or possibly favourable effects on cholesterol, even with its saturated fat content.

On top of its potential effect on blood pressure and cholesterol, cocoa might also improve endothelial function, or the health of the lining of our arteries.[41] The effect seems to be triggered by its flavanol content, particularly through compounds known as catechins.[42] Flavanols are thought to increase production of nitric oxide, or NO, that dandy little compound known to increase vasodilation, allowing more blood flow to the arteries. We'll get into this more in the section on beets, but for now, it's worth mentioning that low levels of NO are associated not only with heart disease but also with erectile dysfunction in men. It might not be surprising, then, to know that Mexico's King Montezuma was given cups of cocoa to drink before he "visited" his wives.[43]

EATING COCOA

The problem with putting cocoa on a superfood list is that it inevitably leads to images of chasing your grass-fed steak and kale dinner with a chocolate cake. When made in the purest sense—from raw cocoa—dark chocolate should, in theory, be rich in flavanols and other disease-fighting nutrients, but the process of making chocolate shares many similarities with the process of making wheat flour: Although the original form of the food is deeply nutritious, once it has been processed, it loses much of what made it so special. In the case of chocolate, the cocoa is often fermented or alkalized when it is turned into chocolate, which can destroy some of those healthy flavanols that are thought to provide much of the health benefit. In a review of the effects of cocoa and chocolate, published by the Center for Science in the Public Interest in *Nutrition Action Healthletter*, to obtain the 200 mg of flavanols required to see a significant effect on blood flow, you would need to eat either 300 grams of milk chocolate (about the equivalent of six chocolate bars), 55 grams of dark chocolate (about the amount in one chocolate bar—assuming the cocoa hadn't been processed enough to destroy the flavanols), or 13 grams of (intensely bitter) baking chocolate.[44] Your best bet? Adding 1 3/4 tablespoons of pure cocoa powder, which provides the necessary flavanols in a 20-calorie serving, to your coffee or warm milk.

THE BOTTOM LINE

Cocoa is one of those foods that divide the medical and nutrition community. There are those who argue that chocolate is simply a treat and that any redeeming nutritional value from the cocoa is trivial compared with the sugar and saturated fats found in a typical chocolate bar. No doubt, some people may use cocoa's nutrition profile as an excuse to indulge, as is often the case with red wine. Although it's true that cocoa corrupted into a plastic-y candy bar is probably going to trigger more heart attacks than it prevents, pure cocoa seems to, at worst, have a neutral effect on our health, but at best, its mineral content, fibre, and flavanol content suggest that—and research doesn't disagree—the notion that it is a food of the gods has some merit. The key, of course, is finding a way to include cocoa in your diet in the purest form possible. And that may well be an acquired taste.

EGGS

Eggs have been on the nutrition rollercoaster for decades. Eschewed in the low-fat diet era for their high cholesterol content, eggs gradually made their way back onto our plates as research increasingly called into question the link between dietary cholesterol and heart disease. But that's not to say the debate is over: In a well-publicized 2010 review, published in the *Canadian Journal of Cardiology*, a trio of Canadian researchers, including Dr. David Jenkins, the lead researcher on the portfolio diet for cholesterol control, lashed out at medical and nutrition professionals for recommending eggs to those at risk for cardiovascular disease. Their conclusion? "Stopping the consumption of egg yolks after a stroke or myocardial infarction [heart attack] would be like quitting smoking after a diagnosis of lung cancer: a necessary action, but late."[45] Damning words, to be sure, but are they fair? Let's take a closer look.

EGGS: THE STORY

According to *Encyclopedia Britannica*, eggs are "the content of the hard-shelled reproductive body produced by a bird, considered as food." The primary function of an egg is to provide both the environment and nutrients for a bird to develop and eventually hatch. Commercial eggs, however, are not fertilized, and as such, no matter how long you might choose to sit on them, they will never hatch. Although the eggs of numerous species, including ducks, geese, quail, and turkey, are produced and used for food around the world, chicken eggs are the most commonly available egg in North America.

The edible part of the egg is divided into two parts: the yolk, which is usually yellow and rich in fats and fat-soluble nutrients, and the white, which is often clear when the egg is uncooked and is composed primarily of protein.

EGGS: THE NUTRITION

One large (50 gram) egg provides 71 calories' worth of energy, along with 5 grams of fat, of which 2 grams are saturated, the type of fat that has been associated (increasingly controversially) with heart disease. According to Health Canada's guidelines, healthy adults should aim to consume less than 20 grams of saturated fat per day, which means two eggs would provide about a fifth of your "bad" fats for the day. But more concerning is the 211 mg of cholesterol per egg, an amount just shy of the 250 mg-per-day limit, also recommended by Health Canada.

So, where is the good news? That same large egg provides 6 grams of high-quality protein (roughly 3 grams each from the yolk and the white), along with 5% of your daily vitamin A, 14% of your riboflavin (vitamin B_2), and 11% of your vitamin B_{12} needs for the day. You'll also obtain 5% of your iron and an impressive 23% of your selenium for the day. Double that portion to two whole eggs and you'll obtain more than 10% of your daily requirements for vitamins A, B_2, folate, vitamin B_{12}, iron, phosphorus, and selenium, along with 12 grams of protein. As a source of protein and fat, eggs also have virtually no effect on blood sugar.

Egg yolks, the controversial part of the egg where the fat, and specifically cholesterol, is stored, are also one of the best-known common food sources of the nutrients lutein and zeaxanthin, both of which have been associated with eye health.[46] Eggs are also a rich source of choline, a nutrient that helps build acetylcholine, a neurotransmitter that is important for healthy nerve and brain function.

Egg whites have long been a popular choice for weight- and cholesterol-conscious individuals. With the yolk removed, egg whites are naturally fat free and, as a consequence, contain no cholesterol (cholesterol is a type of fat in animal foods and also a fat that circulates in the bloodstream). At 16 calories per white, the caloric savings are substantial: two eggs provide 142 calories' worth of energy, but two egg whites provide a mere 32 calories. Of course, you're getting a lot less food with two whites, including less protein (you're tossing away about 3 grams of protein every time you ditch a yolk). You also lose much of the vitamin and mineral content, including all of the vitamins A, D, E, B_{12}, and folate; all of the iron, lutein, and zeaxanthin; and most of the selenium and choline whenever you wash the yellow stuff down the drain or toss it in your compost bin.

Although the data provided here is derived from the USDA database (the Canadian Nutrient File also has similar data), some egg producers contend that their eggs are exceptionally nutrient rich. According to Burnbrae Farms, the makers of Naturegg Omega Pro eggs, one of their large eggs provide substantially more vitamin A (10% vs. 5%), vitamin D (25% vs. 4%), vitamin E (50% vs. 2%), niacin (8% vs. 0%), folate (30% vs. 6%), vitamin B_{12} (80% vs. 11%), and selenium (35% vs. 23%) than traditional eggs.[47] These eggs are also higher in omega-3 fatty acids (see the sidebar Are Omega-3 Eggs Worth It?). Why the difference? It's the feed, don't you know: The hens are fed flaxseed and fish oil, which provide the omega-3 content, and corn, which is responsible for the eggs' high lutein content.

ARE OMEGA-3 EGGS WORTH IT?

It is said that omega-3 eggs were first developed by a Canadian researcher looking to build a healthier egg, especially after all the bad press about their cholesterol content. By feeding hens flaxseed, which is a source of alpha-linolenic acid, or ALA, a plant form of omega-3 fatty acids, the eggs they produced were richer in omega-3s than their traditional counterparts.[48] Unfortunately, since the hens were able to convert only a fraction of the ALA to DHA (the same goes for humans), the omega-3 fatty acid that is considered the most important to human health, this meant the eggs were rich in ALA yet contained only a few milligrams of DHA; by comparison, a serving of oily fish, such as salmon, contains approximately 1,500 to 2,000 mg of DHA. To address this issue, some makers of omega-3 eggs, including Burnbrae Farms, the producers of Naturegg Omega Pro eggs, add fish oil to the chickens' feed, resulting in an egg that provides 125 mg of DHA. Although that is hardly comparable to the amount of DHA in oily fish, it does mean that two eggs provide 250 mg of DHA, only slightly less than a serving of white fish, such as tuna or cod. The bottom line? If you don't eat fish, then omega-3 eggs could be an option, but it's worth bearing in mind that harvesting fish for fish oils can cost the environment; if you do eat oily fish regularly (typical recommendations are twice per week), however, then you're better off to skip the omega-3 eggs and save your money for good-quality eggs from your local farmers' market.

EGGS: THE SCIENCE

One of the first landmark studies to examine the relationship between egg consumption and cardiovascular health was published in 1999 by a group of researchers from the Harvard School of Public Health.[49] The study used data from two large prospective cohort studies: the Health Professionals Follow-Up Study, which followed more than 37,000 men for 18 years, and the Nurses' Health Study, which followed more than 80,000 women for 14 years. At the end of the studies, the incidence of coronary heart disease (CHD) was compared with egg consumption in the diet. After controlling for possible confounding factors, including smoking, age, and other CHD risk factors, the researchers "found no evidence of an overall significant association between egg consumption and risk of CHD or stroke in either men or women." The only subgroup that seemed to be affected by eggs were people with type 2 diabetes, who saw their risk of CHD double in men and increase by 50% in women when they consumed an average of seven eggs per week or more.

EGGS AND SALMONELLA

One of the biggest risks associated with eating eggs is foodborne illness, more commonly known as food poisoning. According to the U.S. Centers for Disease Control and Prevention (CDC), eggs were responsible for more outbreaks of foodborne illness from 2009 to 2010 than any other commodity.[50] The main culprit is usually salmonella, and although Health Canada claims it is not very common in Canadian eggs, it is still important to take appropriate precautions. Salmonella can be particularly dangerous for people with reduced immune capacity, including the elderly, young children and babies, pregnant woman, and individuals with compromised immune systems. To reduce the risk of contracting salmonella, or any other foodborne illness from eggs, be sure to wash your hands thoroughly with soap and warm water for 20 seconds after handling eggs. All utensils and food preparation surfaces and containers should also be thoroughly cleaned. Hard-boiled eggs can be kept in their shell in the refrigerator for up to a week, but any egg that has been left at room temperature (or above) for more than two hours should be discarded. When shopping for eggs, avoid eggs that are cracked or broken or that stick to the bottom of the egg carton. If you are preparing a food that calls for raw or undercooked eggs, such as mayonnaise, Caesar salad dressing, ice cream, or eggnog, it is recommended that you purchase pasteurized eggs to reduce your risk.[51]

Several other cohort studies have been published since the Harvard study, with largely similar results. In 2007, U.S. researchers published a study examining the relationship between egg consumption and risk of dying from cardiovascular disease in nearly 10,000 adults followed for 20 years.[52] After adjusting for known cardiovascular risk factors, such as age, gender, race, cigarette smoking, and diabetes, the researchers found no relationship in stroke or heart disease risk between those who consumed less than one egg per week and those who consumed more than six eggs per week. Once again, however, when they examined people with diabetes as a subgroup, they did find that those who ate the most eggs (more than six per week) had roughly twice the risk of coronary artery (a.k.a. heart) disease than those who consumed the least.

Likewise, the Physicians' Health Study, which followed 21,000 physicians for 20 years, found that egg consumption was not associated with risk of heart attack or stroke, though in this case, they did find a 23% increased risk of mortality in those who ate seven or more eggs per week—but that group, once again, included people with type 2 diabetes, who might have dragged the average up. Finally, the Health, Aging, and Body Composition (Health ABC) Study, which followed 1,941 older men and women for 9 years, found an association between egg consumption and CVD risk only for older adults with type 2 diabetes.[53]

So why all the fuss? Much of it stems from studies demonstrating that when all else in the diet is kept constant, eggs do, in fact, trigger an increase in total and LDL cholesterol. This relationship seems to be especially strong when a person has a low intake of animal fats to begin with; for example, studies on vegetarians have demonstrated a greater jump in cholesterol levels when they add an egg per day to their diets.

And what about those with diabetes? A group of Australian researchers conducted a randomized controlled trial to examine the direct effect of eating two eggs per day on people with type 2 diabetes who ate a lower-carbohydrate, higher-protein diet. Instead of the customary Western diet of roughly 55% carbohydrate, 30% fat, and 15% protein, for four weeks the 65 subjects were fed a reduced-calorie diet that provided 40% of their calories from carbohydrate, 30% from fat, and 30% from protein (notably, these numbers mimic the dietary recommendations from *The Zone Diet* by Dr. Barry Sears). At the beginning of the study, half the subjects were told to eat two eggs per day, while the other half consumed 100 grams (about 3.5 ounces) of lean meat. Translation? The egg group consumed about 590 mg of cholesterol per day, while the lean-meat group averaged only 213 mg of cholesterol per day. After four weeks on their respective diets, both groups had a "washout" period, whereby they ate their usual diets, and then the groups switched diets so that the egg group ate lean protein and the lean-protein group switched to two eggs per day. This study design is called a crossover study, meaning the subjects cross over between both the control (lean protein diet) and the intervention (high egg diet), ideally in random order. Studies such as this allow subjects to act as their own controls so that researchers do not have to seek out and study an entirely separate group of controls.

At the end of the study, the subjects had lost an average of 6 kg (13.2 pounds), and their LDL ("bad") cholesterol was unchanged compared with the start of the study. Their fasting blood sugar, fasting insulin, and blood pressure all improved, however, as did factors associated with cholesterol, including apolipoprotein B, the protein associated with small, dense LDL. But, most important, there was no difference in any of these values when the subjects consumed eggs or lean meat daily. In other words, consuming 14 eggs per week seemed to have no harmful effect on heart health in people with type 2 diabetes who were losing weight, at least over a four-week period.[54] What would happen if these same individuals continued to eat two eggs a day for a year, or two, or ten? That is something we simply don't know.

In a summary on the effects of eggs on heart health, Harvard School of Public Health researchers Drs. Frank Hu, JoAnn Manson, and Walter C. Willett suggested that eggs' apparent lack of harmful effects on heart health suggests that the other nutrients in eggs may somehow mitigate the effect of the cholesterol. "These findings . . . suggest that among healthy men and women, moderate egg consumption can be part of a nutritious and balanced diet," stated Hu and colleagues in their 2001 paper on the subject. "These results also illustrate the danger of judging health effects of a food by single nutrients or components contained in the food."[55]

DOES CHOLESTEROL CAUSE HEART DISEASE?

There is a long-standing theory that eating cholesterol-rich foods increases the amount of cholesterol circulating in your bloodstream. This theory has, at least in part, formed the basis of recommendations to avoid, or limit, cholesterol-rich foods, including egg yolks and shrimp. But what does the research say? According to the Health ABC Study, dietary cholesterol intake was associated with CVD risk only in older adults with type 2 diabetes. Among that population, those with the highest intake of dietary cholesterol had about three-and-a-half times the risk of developing CVD over a nine-year period versus those with the lowest intake of dietary cholesterol.[56] Other well-controlled studies have suggested that dietary cholesterol can raise total and LDL cholesterol, but the effects are relatively small: For example, keeping saturated fat, total fat, and cholesterol within recommended limits, versus the amounts typically eaten in the American diet, was expected to reduce LDL cholesterol by only 5%.[57]

Although there is growing consensus that we need to rethink our view of dietary fats and heart disease (with an emphasis on controlling carbohydrate intake, especially refined grains and added sugars, while emphasizing nutrient-rich whole foods), the story of eggs—and beef, and cheese—can still rankle many. It is always worth bearing in mind, however, that the possibility of confirmation bias exists, even among scientists and researchers. Confirmation bias occurs when we like something (usually a theory, rationale, or argument), leading us to agree with any new information that confirms our belief. In the world of nutrition, that might mean not only celebrating studies that confirm our belief but also consciously or unconsciously overlooking flaws in research that might be contrary to our theory. Likewise, if we read or hear something that goes against the narrative we have created, we are quick to dismiss it, or we pull it to pieces until we find enough problems that we can feel our theory is still safe. Confirmation bias is, at its core, a part of human nature; it frames how we see other people, view belief systems different from ours, and, ultimately, sleep peacefully at night, knowing that the world around us is as it should be. At the end of the day, it's a lower-stress way of living.

This is the crux of why well-controlled studies are so important to help us get to the bottom of a nutrition issue or problem; without carefully crafted measures such as blinding (making sure the subjects, and the researchers, are unaware of who is receiving the treatment versus who is receiving the placebo), conscious and, perhaps more important, unconscious bias can creep in. And that brings us back to the ongoing debate about eggs: If you took two absolute experts on either side of the subject and bought them lunch, there's a better than average chance you'd end up with at least one empty chair by the time the first round of cocktails was finished. And that's where things stand with eggs, at least until one team manages to wiggle more people out of their comfort zone and onto their side, which, if you have studied human nature, you know is not easy to do.

THE BOTTOM LINE

Eggs have a well-deserved place on the superfood controversy list. With a nutrition profile that other foods would envy (if they could), eggs seem like a great addition to most any diet. But with questions about the effect of eggs on cholesterol levels and heart disease risk, especially for people with diabetes, still lingering, a number of questions about eggs remain unanswered. For now, however, the idea of eating eggs in moderation, as part of a healthy diet, does not seem unreasonable; in more time, we might be able to swing the pendulum more decisively one way or the other.

PEANUT BUTTER

Once a lunchtime staple, peanut butter has tumbled down the nutrition ladder, not only because of its high fat and calorie content but also because of its potential to trigger severe food allergies. Poor public image aside, however, peanut butter actually boasts an impressive nutrition résumé: It is one of the relatively few foods rich in vitamin E, and research demonstrates that regular nut and nut-butter consumers tend to have an easier time controlling their body weight than their nut-avoiding counterparts. Although this seems counterintuitive—after all, nuts and nut butters are among the highest-calorie foods around—nuts may help with weight control by serving as natural appetite suppressors, and research suggests that some of the calories from nuts end up being excreted in our waste. What's more, with a health food craze that has us shelling out big bucks for the latest berry imported from Outer Mongolia, peanut butter remains one of the cheapest and most portable superfoods around.

PEANUT BUTTER: THE STORY

You might have heard that peanuts are not actually a nut but instead are a legume. In fact, peanuts (*Arachis hypogaea*) are derived from the same Fabaceae, or pea, family as the likes of lentils and chickpeas. Unlike their leguminous cousins, however, peanuts ripen underground. Native to South America, peanuts are now cultivated in the United States, China, West Africa, and India and grow well in many warm or tropical climates.

Virtually unheard of in the United States at the turn of the 20th century, peanuts were brought to the forefront of American culture by an agricultural scientist named George Washington Carver.[211] Born in Missouri to a slave mother, Carver was freed as a child during the U.S. Civil War, but he ended up returning, frail and sick, to the plantation where he was born. Although he was no longer a slave, Carver remained on the plantation, where he developed a strong interest in plants and animals and eventually received an education, culminating in a master of science degree in 1896.

As a native of the U.S. South, Carver was keenly aware of the devastation to farmland from the decades of relentless cotton production. He proposed, as a means of returning the soil to health, the cultivation of both soybeans and peanuts, two crops that add nitrogen back to the soil, which could also serve as a source of protein for many undernour-ished Southerners.

Despite Carver's best efforts, there was little demand for these then-uncommon foods. Undaunted, however, Carver took it upon himself to conduct research on the potential uses for both peanuts and sweet potatoes, another food well suited to the soil of the region. By the end of his career, Carver had developed some 300 products from peanuts, ranging from edible products, such as cheeses, coffee, and flour, to inks, dyes, stains, medicinal oils, and cosmetics (he also developed more than a hundred products from sweet potatoes). With Carver's efforts, it is perhaps not surprising that the peanut soon became a boom product for U.S. farmers: By the mid-1900s, it had become one of the top six crops in the United States and was the second-most valuable crop in the South.

PEANUT BUTTER: THE NUTRITION

A 2-tablespoon (32 gram) serving of peanut butter has an attractive nutrition profile, providing some 188 calories' worth of energy along with 7 grams of protein, 2 grams of fibre, and 16 grams of fat, of which nearly 7 grams are monounsaturated, one of the types of fat that tends to be associated with heart health. A serving of peanut butter also pro-vides 10% of your daily value for vitamin E, which, although lower than almonds, is still among the top food sources of the hard-to-get vitamin, along with 21% of your niacin (vitamin B_3) and 9% of your vitamin B_6 needs for the day. Among minerals, peanut butter is particularly rich in selenium, providing 18% of your daily needs, along with 14% of your magnesium, 6% of your zinc, and 5% of your potassium. All in all, aside from the vitamin E content, peanut butter's nutrition is actually quite similar to that of another perceived nutrition superstar, almonds.

PEANUT BUTTER: THE SCIENCE
Peanut Butter and Weight

As mentioned, peanuts and peanut butter seem to have a natural appetite-suppressing effect that could translate into weight loss. But is one form of peanut better than the other? Researchers from Brazil took up the challenge of comparing peanuts to peanut butter in a study on 15 women at high risk of developing type 2 diabetes.[59] In the study, they gave the women an equal serving of peanuts or peanut butter—or neither—in a carbohydrate-based breakfast and tracked the women's blood sugar and appetite hormone response for the next four hours. Since we know that fats, fibre, and protein (all of which are found in peanuts and peanut butter) are more satiating (filling) than carbohydrate foods that are low in fibre, it is not surprising that the subjects' blood sugars were significantly lower; their appetite-suppressing hormones, including cholecystokinin (CCK) and peptide YY (PYY), were higher; and their desire to eat was lower after eating the peanut butter–based breakfast versus the control (carbohydrate only) breakfast. What was surprising, however, was that the same effect was not observed with whole peanuts. Although the peanuts did trigger positive trends, these trends weren't strong enough to reach statistical significance, suggesting that for some reason peanut butter might be more filling than its whole counterpart.

And what of the effect of peanut butter on weight? No doubt a high-calorie food, the image of the dumped girlfriend soothing herself with a jar of peanut butter has left many of us with the impression that it is as fattening as it comes. And while no one is going to recommend using ladles full of peanut butter for weight loss, it is intriguing to see studies, such as one in 2010 by researchers at Purdue University, demonstrate that a daily dose of 56 grams of peanuts (either raw, roasted, salted, unsalted, or even honey roasted) or peanut butter for four weeks had no effect on body weight in 118 overweight or obese adults.[60] It did, however, help improve the cardiovascular profile of those who already had high cholesterol, by bringing down total and LDL ("bad") cholesterol as well as triglycerides.

Peanut Butter and Heart Health

So, at least one study demonstrated that peanut butter could help bring cholesterol down, but are there others? In 1999, well-known nutrition scientist Penny Kris-Etherton and a team of researchers at Penn State University and the University of Rochester examined the effect of the standard cholesterol-lowering diet, known as the National Cholesterol Education Program (NCEP) Step II diet, versus a diet higher in monounsaturated fats from either olive oil or peanuts and peanut butter.[61] All three diets were compared with a control diet mimicking the average American diet. The Step II diet, which is designed to help people with high cholesterol reduce their risk of heart attack or stroke, is low in fat (providing about 25% of calories from fat; the average American diet provides about 35%), saturated fat, and cholesterol. Interestingly, however, the olive oil and peanut/peanut butter diets in the study were designed not to mimic the Step II diet; instead they provided as much total fat as the average American consumes but substituted olive oil or peanuts and peanut butter for the saturated and trans fats that Americans tend to eat. All the diets were designed to keep the participants' weight stable, so the results should have been due to the changes in the composition of the various diets, not due to weight loss.

The results probably raised a few eyebrows at the time. Although all three intervention diets (the Step II, the olive oil, and the peanut/peanut butter diets) reduced LDL ("bad") cholesterol versus the average American diet, the Step II diet sent a few measures in the wrong direction. Versus the average American diet, the Step II diet not only *lowered* HDL ("good") cholesterol but also *raised* triglycerides, a type of fat that circulates in the bloodstream that can be harmful to our hearts. We now understand that the reason for these seemingly oddball results is that a low-fat diet often goes hand in hand with eating more carbohydrate, and it's usually not the good kind. Back in the 1990s, when this study was conducted, cutting down on fats didn't mean eating more quinoa or lentils; instead it meant more white rice, pasta, bagels, and low-fat (but high-sugar) desserts, such as frozen yogurt. These foods are low in nutritional value, and they cause a spike in blood sugar and insulin after eating them, leaving us feeling more hungry. The blood sugar fluctuations can also cause our triglycerides to rise. In other words, cutting down fat is one thing, but if you replace the fats with low-quality carbohydrate foods, you might just be worse off than before. Fast forward 15 years or so, and we now have a much greater appreciation that the low-fat diet craze probably did more harm than good, and the blood work of these subjects is one piece of evidence.

So, what happened to the peanut/peanut butter and olive oil groups? The participants on both diets rich in monounsaturated fat saw only their LDL cholesterol drop; their HDL and triglycerides went in the right directions—and all of that while on a diet with 35% of their calories from fat. The final punchline? When the researchers calculated the subjects' risk of developing cardiovascular disease, the olive oil and peanut/peanut butter groups saw their risk drop by 25% and 21%, respectively, while the Step II diet yielded only a 12% decline. To make a long story short: Peanut butter might be a high-calorie food, but if you include it in your diet instead of whatever you grabbed from Starbucks this afternoon, it could go a long way to improving your overall health.

CAN PEANUT ALLERGIES BE CURED?

No doubt, allergy is the biggest concern when it comes to peanuts and peanut butter. Food allergy is estimated to affect nearly 4% of children in industrialized countries, and peanut allergy seems to be on the rise. Why are we seeing more allergies in kids? We don't know for sure, but some possibilities include the "hygiene theory" (the notion that children are not exposed to enough environmental challenges—such as dirt—early in life, which sets up their immune systems to overrespond when they are exposed to foreign substances later on), inadequate vitamin D exposure (it affects the way our immune system works), and differences in the way peanuts are processed (for example, boiled peanuts, which are more common in Asia, where peanut allergy tends to be lower, may be easier for our bodies to break down than roasted peanuts, which are served more commonly in North America, and therefore enter the bloodstream as smaller, and better tolerated, proteins).

Regardless of origin, the treatment for peanut allergy remains the same: strict avoidance for life. That is, until some recent forays into a treatment known as oral immunotherapy, or OIT, started to pique the interest of the allergic masses (a group that, for what it's worth, includes this author). OIT is founded on the notion of giving a small dose of allergen, in this case, peanut flour, and increasing that dose gradually until symptoms are observed. In this process, patients do reach the point of having enough of an allergic reaction that they feel a bit uncomfortable. That threshold of feeling just a bit of an allergic response is then set as the starting point for the therapy, after which small amounts of the peanut flour are given daily for several months, until a reasonable amount of tolerance is achieved.

To date, the best trial on OIT was published in the *Journal of Allergy and Clinical Immunology* in 2011.[62] In this study, a team of physicians and researchers at the University of Arkansas and Duke University gave a group of 28 children, ranging in age from 1 to 16 years old, a gradually increasing dose of peanut flour, starting from a baseline of at least 1.5 mg (that's 0.0015 grams) of peanut protein and eventually working up to 5,000 mg, or the equivalent of 20 peanuts, in one sitting. The process took about a year. Although those in the peanut group did experience some side effects (three subjects had to drop out early because of allergic responses), those who remained eventually saw their allergies, measured through skin prick and lab tests, improve significantly versus the nine control patients, who also had peanut allergy but consumed gradually increasing amounts of oat flour, rather than peanut flour, throughout the study.

Although the results of the study will no doubt provide a ray of hope for families suffering with peanut allergies, there is still plenty of reason for caution: The study excluded any child with a history of life-threatening peanut allergy, with moderate to severe asthma, or with uncontrolled eczema. In other words, while OIT may have potential benefit for some individuals with peanut allergy, it is still not recommended for those in the greatest danger. In fact, a review conducted by the *Cochrane Database of Systematic Reviews*, which highlighted the Arkansas/Duke study in the analysis, concluded that "in view of the risk of adverse events and the lack of evidence of long-term benefits, allergen-specific peanut OIT cannot currently be recommended as a treatment for the management of patients with IgE-mediated peanut allergy."[63] In other words, until we learn more about this new therapy, we would be well advised to exercise caution.

THE BOTTOM LINE

Eating peanut butter might feel like a social taboo in this day and age, but that doesn't mean we should ditch it altogether (and, for the record, I say this as a person with a peanut allergy). It's simply too rare to find foods with wide-ranging nutrition profiles that are tasty, easy to use, don't require refrigeration, and cost next to nothing. Of course, before we get too excited, we should remember that the reference serving sizes use *level* measuring spoons, not the heaping soup spoons that are so easy to enjoy. So, although a tablespoon or two is reasonable for many individuals (those with high energy needs, such as athletes, can often enjoy more), it's important not to turn this into an excuse to eat peanut butter by the bucket.

POTATOES

If you're going to lose weight and be healthy, you have to take a pass on potatoes, right? Relegated to nutritional Siberia in recent years, white potatoes, unlike their orange-fleshed sweet cousins, are perceived as unhealthy because of their purported impact on blood sugar, which in turn triggers the production of insulin. As the theory goes, when blood sugars run too high for too long, the body's capacity to respond to insulin declines, leading to a condition known as insulin resistance. As the body becomes more insulin resistant, blood sugars drift higher, even in the fasted state, with the end result being the potential development of type 2 diabetes. In addition, foods that cause a spike in blood sugar also tend to produce an inflammatory response in the body, which is thought to be a catalyst for a wide range of illness and disease, ranging from hardened arteries to joint pain to plaques in the brain that are consistent with the onset of Alzheimer's. So, foods that cause a blood sugar and insulin spike, such as white potatoes, have been crossed off many healthy eating lists because of these potential downstream effects. And, when you add to that a number of studies that have demonstrated a correlation between potato consumption and obesity, you might start to wonder what the heck potatoes are doing in a book on superfoods.

POTATOES: THE STORY

Potatoes (*Solanum tuberosum*) are a tuberous food crop made up of the swollen ends of the stolon, or underground stem of the potato plant. Potatoes have a long and volatile history of use in many parts of the world. Originally found in South America, potatoes tolerate altitude better than most edible plant foods, which made them a hardy staple for those living in and around the Andes Mountains. Potatoes were eventually brought to Europe by the Spanish, who also coined the name "batata," in the 16th century. In both Europe and North America, their adoption was slowed because of concerns by puritanical groups that they were not mentioned in the Bible. Over time, however, potatoes evolved into a staple food and helped save both the Irish and Prussians from famine in the 1700s. From 1845 to 1849, however, late blight, a fungal infection, destroyed the Irish potato harvest for multiple years, leading to a famine that killed a million people and led to the emigration of two million more.

POTATOES: THE NUTRITION

For all their controversy, it might surprise you to learn that a medium (173 gram) baked potato, with the skin on, provides 4 grams of fibre, 4 grams of protein, and just 161 calories—only a couple of calories higher than an equal-sized serving of sweet potato—along with 28% of your daily vitamin C (yes, vitamin C) needs and 27% of your vitamin B_6, a nutrient involved in more than a hundred reactions in the human body, especially in the development of healthy brain cells. Potatoes also provide 10% of your daily iron; 12% each of your vitamin B_3, folate, and magnesium needs; and a whopping 26%, or 926 mg, of your potassium needs (that's three times the amount in a banana)—making it, along with sweet potatoes, the richest source of potassium of any commonly consumed food.

But, herein lies the rub. As soon as you take the skin off the potato, the nutritional value drops: A medium boiled, skinless potato still provides 21% of your daily vitamin C needs but only 3% of your iron, 4% of your folate, and 16% of your potassium (548 mg). It also makes your blood sugar rise more precipitously. And if you fry the potato, not only will the calories jump, but you will also get a dose of acryl-amide, a compound that has carcinogenic effects in rats, which is produced when potatoes and other starchy foods are cooked at very high temperatures.[64] In other words, when it comes to potatoes, it's best to leave the jacket on.

POTATOES: THE SCIENCE

Despite their impressive nutrition profile, potatoes have not always fared well in the world of research. For example, several studies have linked Western meat-and-potatoes diets, which feature potatoes as a staple food, to an increased risk of colorectal adenoma or cancer.[65,66] Fried potatoes have also been associated with higher fasting blood sugar and insulin levels in large cohort studies.[67] The problem, of course, is that potatoes in all forms are also often grouped together for research purposes, which means that baked or roasted potatoes with the skin on are found in the same category as potato chips and French fries. As a result, it can be difficult to determine just how well (or poorly) potatoes can fit in a healthy diet. Potatoes, like full-fat dairy and beef, are also often lumped in the research with low-nutrient diets or lifestyles that have been associated with disease risk: No doubt, a hamburger with fries and a pop would have a different effect on your health than a baked potato with a salmon filet and a spinach salad.

As a result of the conflict between potatoes' nutritional value and their negative public image, a handful of studies and reviews have recently been published that re-examine the role potatoes do play in our health.[68] In an analysis of data from the National Health and Nutrition Examination Survey (NHANES), for example, it was found that potato consumers tended to eat more total vegetables and had higher potassium intakes than non-consumers (note that, in this study, potatoes were considered separately from French fries).[69] Potatoes also contributed nearly a quarter of the dietary fibre and 20% of potassium for teens but represented only 11% of their energy (calorie) intake. (It should be noted, however, that this analysis of the data was conducted by researchers from the Alliance for Potato Research and Education in McLean, Virginia.)

The potassium content in potatoes is also of great significance. Potassium has been dubbed a "shortfall nutrient" in the United States, meaning it is often underconsumed. Potassium plays an important role in blood pressure control, and it also may protect against bone loss as we age and might even help prevent kidney stones.[70] Because meeting the recommended 4,700 mg of potassium per day is a challenge for many (remember, a banana contains about 300 mg), emphasizing a whole-foods diet that includes a variety of potassium-rich foods, such as fruits, vegetables, and, yes, potatoes is necessary to reach the target.

And what about potatoes and blood sugar? Here there is also a story. Despite the image that potatoes have a huge effect on blood sugar, research looking at the glycemic index (blood-sugar-raising effect) of potatoes has produced mixed results, with some studies finding potatoes have a low GI and some high. Part of the variation could stem from the way the potato is prepared (skin on versus peeled; boiled versus baked) as well as the variability between different types of potatoes, but the bottom line is that, in moderate portions, potatoes don't necessarily send blood sugar as haywire as we might have been led to believe.

Potatoes have also earned a bad reputation because of a belief that they trigger an insulin response greater than any other fruit or vegetable (insulin response to food is usually, but not always, related to the food's effect on blood sugar). Once again, the facts differ from the legend: In a study by Australian researchers on what is now known as the insulin index (a measure of a food's ability to trigger an insulin response compared with white bread), potatoes initially seemed to have a massive effect on insulin levels and were one of the few foods to generate an overall insulin score higher than white bread.[71] There is, however, a catch: Because the researchers used 240-calorie portions for each food, they had to use the equivalent of about two medium potatoes—a portion size up to four times larger than some other calorie-rich foods (and they peeled and boiled them, too, which means a good chunk of the fibre was lost). As a result, potatoes came out looking worse than not only white bread but also donuts, croissants, cake, cookies, and even potatoes' arch-enemies, French fries and potato chips. But again, because these foods are high in calories, they used smaller portions, so it's no wonder potatoes fared so poorly!

If, on the other hand, we look at the results *by gram of food*, potatoes actually ended up near the bottom of the pile, producing less of an insulin response than rye bread, brown rice, bananas, and even peanuts, yogurt, and beef. Perhaps not surprisingly (but intriguingly), because the researchers used such a large portion of potatoes, they scored the highest rating for fullness of any food studied, beating out the likes of beef, eggs, brown pasta, peanuts, oatmeal, and fish.[72]

POTATOES: THE CAVEATS

In addition to having concerns about the effects of potatoes on blood sugar and insulin, as well as acrylamide in fried potato products, some individuals avoid potatoes because they belong to the nightshade family. The nightshade family also includes eggplant, bell peppers, cayenne peppers, and tomatoes, and these foods have been anecdotally associated with arthritis and chronic pain. Some people believe that, once they eliminated nightshades, which share a common lineage with some poisonous plants, their symptoms of pain and stiffness improved. To date, no well-controlled studies have demonstrated a link between nightshades and joint pain or inflammation, so it remains a question mark for many.

Potatoes also have the dubious distinction of being on the Environmental Working Group's Dirty Dozen Plus list of produce that is most likely to be contaminated with pesticides.[73] As a result, it is often recommended that you purchase organic potatoes when possible.

When purchasing potatoes, avoid green spots; they indicate the presence of a natural toxin, known as solanine. Although solanine levels in most potatoes are low, they rise dramatically in potatoes that have been exposed to light, which also triggers the change in colour. Solanines also develop in the eyes and sprouts of the potato, so care should be taken to remove these before cooking. To prevent the greening of the potato, as well as the growth of eyes and sprouts, it's important to store potatoes in a cool, dark place rather than on a countertop. Although some solanine may be lost to the water if the potatoes are boiled (which means it's important to avoid reusing potato water if the potatoes had green spots, eyes, or sprouts), it is not deactivated by cooking. Solanine consumption is associated with a bitter taste, a burning sensation in the mouth, stomach upset, nausea, and vomiting.[74]

THE BOTTOM LINE

Potatoes have been much maligned, but perhaps unfairly so. Just as turning lean pork into a hot dog or a fish filet into fish and chips perverts the once-rich nutrition profile, peelers and deep fryers have given potatoes a bad name. So, if you're thinking about reintroducing potatoes into your diet, keep it simple: Buy organic if you can, try roasting or baking with the skin on, and enjoy them as part of a balanced meal.

4

CLASSICS!

SUPERFOODS THAT STILL RULE

So, what have you learned so far? That superfoods can't easily be characterized, sometimes behave unpredictably, and can help eager opportunists earn a pretty penny when consumers jump on the bandwagon. Despite all the confusion, however, there are still some safe bets that almost anyone can benefit from, including in their diet. Almonds, avocados, beans, blueberries: All have lots going for them, and in many cases, we understand their benefits reasonably well. So, what can these foods offer you?

ALMONDS
Almonds have been on the list of superfoods for as long as the term has been used. Once spurned in the low-fat era of the 1980s and 1990s, almonds have made their way back into popular consciousness as research increasingly demonstrated the benefits of so-called good fats.

ALMONDS: THE STORY
Almonds (*Prunis dulcis*) are actually the fruit of a tree that is part of the rose family. In the early stages of growth, you'd be hard pressed

to tell an almond apart from a peach, which happens to be a close relative—that is, until they mature, at which point the almond's outer covering splits open, and out pops the nut. Almonds exist as two varieties: bitter and sweet. Like a number of species from the rose family, bitter almonds contain compounds that are toxic to humans, though they can be refined into almond oil and extracts, such as amaretto, for flavouring and aroma. Sweet almonds, on the other hand, are edible and have enjoyed a long history of human consumption.

ALMONDS: THE NUTRITION

Make no mistake: All nuts, almonds included, are high-calorie foods. But research published by the Almond Board of California, as well as the United States Department of Agriculture, has forced us to rethink their actual versus predicted calorie content. According to traditional models, a 1-ounce (28 gram) serving of almonds, which is the equivalent of 23 whole kernels, should provide about 162 calories' worth of energy. The new data, published in the *American Journal of Clinical Nutrition* in August 2012, however, suggests that almonds contain about 30 fewer calories per serving than initially predicted.[1] That same 1-ounce serving actually provides 129 calories' worth of energy, or about a 20% savings in energy. (Quick! Eat more!)

The discrepancy is believed to relate to something known as the Atwater general factors, which are used to determine the amount of energy in food. Developed more than a hundred years ago by Wilbur Olin Atwater, a chemist at the USDA, the system is still widely used to estimate the amount of calories in a food. At its core, the old system estimated how easily our bodies digested the proteins, carbohydrates, and fats in foods. Those numbers, in turn, could be used to estimate the number of calories the food contained. Although the numbers have been in use for years, evidence began to mount that the fats in whole peanuts and tree nuts (of which almonds are one) were not digested as efficiently as other fats. Instead, it seems that some of the fats pass straight through our digestive systems, at which point they are quite literally flushed down the toilet.

Calories aside, what else do almonds have to offer? Reverting back to the old data for a moment, an ounce of almonds provides 6 grams of protein, 3 grams of fibre, and 14 grams of fat (that number is likely lower, based on the new data). Of the fat, the majority (about 9 grams) is derived from monounsaturated fatty acids, or MUFAs, a type of fat associated with many of the health benefits of the Mediterranean diet. The rest of the fat is largely derived from the omega-6 family of polyunsaturated fats.

Almonds are also an outstanding source of vitamin E. Although research on vitamin E supplements has not panned out, a range of studies suggest that vitamin E status is associated with better cognitive function as we age.[2, 3, 4] Unfortunately, vitamin E is one of the most difficult nutrients to obtain in your diet, especially if you choose only low-fat foods: Many of the best food sources of vitamin E are higher-fat foods, including nuts, seeds, and plant oils (some lower-fat foods, including certain green, leafy vegetables, kiwi, tomato paste and tomato products, and wheat germ also contain vitamin E). It's for this reason that almonds are so appealing: An ounce provides 37% of your daily vitamin E needs, which exceeds almost any other commonly available food.

Aside from healthy fats and vitamin E, almonds are also a good source of magnesium (19% of your daily value) and provide 200 mg of potassium (the adequate intake, or AI, of 4,700 mg is difficult to obtain and requires eating a wide range of potassium-containing foods, such as almonds, throughout the day). Almonds are also a source of calcium, providing 75 mg per serving, which is 7.5% of an average adult's daily needs. They also provide 17% of your daily riboflavin (vitamin B_2) needs, along with 5% of your niacin and 6% of your iron and zinc.

TOP SUPERFOOD SOURCES OF VITAMIN E

FOOD	PORTION	VITAMIN E	VITAMIN E (% DAILY VALUE)
Egg, Omega Pro	1 large	~	50%
Almonds	28.5 g (23 whole almonds)	7.4 mg	37%
Avocado	1 cup, cubed (150 g)	3.1 mg	16%
Kiwi, skinless	2 large (182 g)	2.6 mg	14%
Peanut butter	2 tbsp (32 g)	1.9 mg	10%
Blackberries, raw	1 cup (144 g)	1.7 mg	8%
Sweet potato	1 cup, baked in skin (200 g)	1.4 mg	7%
Quinoa	1 cup, cooked (185 g)	1.2 mg	6%
Raspberries	1 cup (123 g)	1.1 mg	5%

Source: USDA National Nutrient Database (all except egg, retrieved from www.burnbraefarms.com/consumer/our_products/chart_omega_pro.htm)

- = data not available

ALMONDS: THE SCIENCE

Of all the superfoods, almonds have the distinction of being one of the best researched. A number of well-controlled studies, both short and long term, have been conducted on the effects of almonds on their own as well as in conjunction with other healthy foods.

For more than a decade, a Toronto-based research team, led by Dr. David Jenkins, have conducted a series of studies on how a diet that regularly includes almonds can affect heart health and diabetes management. The diet plan, which the researchers dubbed the portfolio diet, or portfolio eating plan, includes 1 to 1.5 ounces (30 to 45 grams) of almonds per day; at least 20 grams of a type of cholesterol-lowering fibre known as soluble, viscous fibre (common sources of soluble fibre, which forms a gel and binds cholesterol in the intestine, include oats, berries, and beans); and soy products and foods fortified with plant sterols, a cholesterol-lowering compound found in plant foods. Some of the studies on the portfolio eating plan have used vegetarian diets, while more recent phases have included moderate portions of meat.

The results of the portfolio diet research have been impressive, to say the least. In one classic study, Dr. Jenkins' team compared their carefully crafted portfolio eating plan to the U.S. National Cholesterol Education Program Step II diet in subjects with elevated cholesterol (as mentioned in the section on peanut butter, the NCEP diet is characterized by its low saturated fat and cholesterol content, while also including low-fat dairy and whole wheat cereals).[5] At the start of the study, one group of subjects was placed on the Step II diet, which was used as the control diet for the study. The second group was introduced to the portfolio diet, while the third group was placed on the Step II diet and also given 20 mg of the cholesterol-lowering drug Lovastatin. The objective of the study was to see what would happen after a month on the portfolio eating plan versus following traditional cholesterol-lowering dietary recommendations, including taking medication.

In many ways, the results of the study changed the way we viewed the potential for diet to control cholesterol. Although the control group on the Step II diet saw their levels of LDL, the so-called bad cholesterol, decline by 8%, and the Step II-plus-Lovastatin group saw their cholesterol drop by 31% (both predictable results, based on what previous studies had shown), the group on the portfolio diet saw their levels of LDL cholesterol drop by 29%, a result close enough to the statin drug that the difference between them was statistically insignificant; in other words, the effects of the statin-drug-plus-Step II diet and the portfolio plan were effectively the same. For the first time, it became apparent that, in the right set of circumstances, dietary change could be just as powerful as medication for the management of high cholesterol.

Beyond cholesterol levels, the statin and portfolio groups also triggered nearly identical 33% and 28% drops in what is known as C-reactive protein (CRP), a measure of inflammation in our bodies that is considered a risk factor for heart disease. Those on the control (Step II only) diet, by comparison, saw their CRP levels drop by only 10%. When all cardiac risk factors were taken together, the statin and portfolio groups reduced their risk of having heart problems, such as a heart attack, stroke, or angina, by about 25% in the 10 years after the study. As for subjects on the Step II diet, their risk dropped by just 3%.

Although the results of these earlier portfolio diet studies were very impressive, our knowledge of heart health has evolved since then. In recent years, research on LDL cholesterol has been taken a step further, as scientists now take into consideration fractions of cholesterol, such as the small, dense LDL that seems to be the most damaging. Well, good news here: In a follow-up study, Dr. Jenkins' research team examined the effect of the portfolio diet on LDL particle size, and the results, once again, were positive: Although the Step II (control) diet brought down small, dense LDL by 0.17 mmol/L, a month on the portfolio eating plan resulted in a drop of 0.69 mmol/L—more than four times the effect of the nationally recognized cholesterol-lowering diet.[6] Although the Step II-plus-statin group experienced the biggest drop in small, dense LDL of all at 0.99 mmol/L, the difference between the statin and portfolio groups did not reach statistical significance, which means that, at least based on these results, the portfolio eating plan was technically no less effective at lowering small, dense LDL than was a diet low in saturated fat and cholesterol coupled with a statin drug.

Now, turning our attention back to almonds: The results of the portfolio studies certainly suggest that almonds are beneficial for heart health, at least when taken as part of a diet that includes other cholesterol-lowering foods. But what about the effect of almonds on their own? Spanish researchers asked this very question when they compared the effects of replacing 40% of fats in the diet with an equal amount of either olive oil, walnuts, or almonds in patients with high cholesterol.[7] After four weeks, the three groups saw their levels of LDL cholesterol drop by 7%, 11%, and 13%, respectively, and the differences between the groups were small enough to be considered statistically insignificant. In other words, this study suggests that almonds can be just as effective as walnuts and olive oil for cholesterol control when used in lieu of unhealthy fats in the diet.

Aside from their impact on cholesterol, almonds also seem to help the body become more sensitive to insulin, which is important for short- and long-term blood sugar control to both prevent and manage type 2 diabetes. In a study comparing the standard American Diabetes Association (ADA) diet with a similar diet that included 2 ounces of almonds per day in 65 adults with prediabetes, U.S. researchers found that in the group who received the almonds, not only did their LDL cholesterol decline, but their insulin levels, measures of insulin resistance, and beta-cell (the part of the pancreas that produces insulin) function all fared better than they did on the traditional ADA diet.[8]

The effect of almonds on blood sugar for people with diabetes can be felt immediately: A smaller study on 19 adults with type 2 diabetes found that an ounce of almonds taken with a breakfast consisting of a bagel, juice, and butter reduced blood sugar by 30% versus eating the meal without almonds.[9] The same researchers also found that eating a single serving of nuts per day, five days per week for 12 weeks, reduced hemoglobin A1c, a measure of average blood sugar levels, by 4%.

Although the research on almonds for heart health and blood sugar control is compelling, there is also a small body of research suggesting that almonds may have a potential benefit for bone health. In a 2011 study, a University of Toronto research team that included Dr. David Jenkins found that consumption of 60 grams (about 2 ounces) of almonds with a mixed meal suppressed markers of bone breakdown, known as osteoclasts (you'll learn more about those in the section on kale), versus an almond-free test meal.[10]

Unfortunately, despite all the evidence we have that almonds are good for our health, many people are still concerned about adding them into their diets out of fear of weight gain because of their high fat content. Fortunately, a 2007 study published in the *British Journal of Nutrition* helped put that fear to bed: In a study conducted by researchers at Purdue University, 20 women were advised to add 50 almonds, or the equivalent of 344 calories' worth, per day to their diets.[11] They were given no other nutrition advice. After 10 weeks, the women who ate the nuts saw no change in their body weight versus controls, even though they hadn't been given any strategies to control their weight. The researchers found that the women who added the almonds to their diets naturally cut back on other foods, which could speak to the appetite-suppressing effects of almonds and other nuts.

ENJOYING YOUR ALMONDS

Although almonds are now available to us in myriad forms, be it as a drink, in bars, or as almond butter, the best way to eat them is the way nature intended: raw, whole, and unsalted. Heating almonds by roasting may cause some of their fats to oxidize (basically, become rancid), though the vitamin E may protect them to a certain degree. To protect the fats in almonds (or any nut), they should be kept in a cool, dry place and should be discarded if they develop an unpleasant smell. Although there is evidence that almonds are perfectly okay for weight control, you should still be mindful not to overdo it: A handful or two per day is plenty for most people.

THE BOTTOM LINE

Whether it's for their protein, fibre, vitamin E, magnesium, calcium, or monounsaturated fat content, there is little argument that almonds are a nutritious choice. What's more, we have good evidence that almonds can help with cholesterol control, reduce inflammation in our bodies, and support blood sugar control for those with diabetes or prediabetes. Perhaps the best news, however, is that they seem to offer all these benefits without causing unwanted weight gain, provided they are eaten in reasonable amounts. It's for all these reasons, and many likely still undiscovered, that almonds have a well-deserved place at the top of any superfood list.

AVOCADOS

Remember "fat makes you fat"? In the 1980s and '90s, we were bombarded with claims that fats were bad for our hearts and our waistlines, and low-fat and fat-free foods permeated the market. So we dropped the fats and instead turned our attention to low-fat candy, crackers, noodles, cookies, and baked goods. We now know this was not the best dietary strategy.

Meanwhile, our collective obsession with cutting out fat meant that a number of highly nutritious foods were banished from our diets for being unhealthy or fattening. Gone were nuts and seeds, olive oil and oily fish, and along with them went the avocado, that oddball fruit with the tough outer layer. High in fat and calories—what a double whammy!—the dark green fruit (yes, it's technically a fruit) has mercifully started to wend its way back now that we have finally begun to truly appreciate its remarkable nutrition profile.

AVOCADOS: THE STORY

A member of the Lauraceae, or laurel family, avocados (*Persea americana*, also known as alligator pear) are a true food of the Americas. With a history that dates back to between 5,000 and 7,000 B.C., wild avocados are believed to have originated in Mexico, but the first evidence of cultivated avocados was in Peru, where they have been found buried with Incan mummies circa 750 B.C.[12] Today, 90% of U.S. avocados are grown in California, where they are harvested year-round. Although Fuerte avocados were for years the top variety in the United States, they have now been replaced by the Hass (often misspelled Haas), a variety of avocado that was patented by Rudolph Hass in 1935. A postman by trade, Hass had the original tree bearing his name in his backyard, and according to Hass Avocados, he was preparing to cut it down when his children, who preferred the taste of Hass's avocados over any other, talked him out of it.[13]

Avocados are typically best enjoyed raw or in uncooked prepared dishes, such as guacamole. Although avocados may be quite hard when purchased, they do ripen at room temperature, eventually resulting in a deep purple to black skin that yields to gentle pressure. To open an avocado, simply use a sharp knife to slice it lengthwise, being mindful to cut around the large, smooth pit in the middle. Gently twisting the avocado around the pit should allow it to separate nicely. From there, you can scoop the flesh out with a spoon or cut it out with a knife. As for the half of the avocado that still has the pit, you can use the same knife to grab it with a single sharp chop (this requires a bit of confidence). As long as the knife is well secured in the pit, a bit of wiggling should pull it right out.

Although guacamole is probably the quintessential avocado-based dish, avocados have far more to offer in the kitchen. Cubed avocados make great additions to salads and do particularly well with the likes of black beans, corn, red onions, lime, and cilantro. Although it might seem strange, avocados also make terrific additions to smoothies, adding a lovely buttery thickness that makes your drink seem decadent. Avocados also work wonders with wraps, burgers, and sandwiches, either in slices as a topper or as a spread in lieu of butter or mayonnaise.

AVOCADOS: THE NUTRITION

You could make the case that avocados are perhaps the most nutritionally well-rounded fruit or vegetable. A cup of cubed raw avocado (150 grams), equal to about three-quarters of a whole avocado, provides 10 grams of fibre—that's 40% of the daily needs for an average female, and more than you'd get from a 1/2-cup serving of beans—along with a quarter of your vitamin C, 16% of the hard-to-get antioxidant vitamin E, and 39% of your vitamin K requirements (to be fair, a cup is double the serving size in Canada's Food Guide, so dividing all those numbers in half will make them look, well, half as good). You'll also pick up more than 10% of most of your B vitamins, along with a hefty 30% of your folate needs, which means that avocados make a great choice for women who are looking to become pregnant (folate, the natural form of folic acid, a B vitamin, is known to reduce the risk of neural tube defects in the unborn fetus). A cup of avocado also provides more than 10% of your daily value for magnesium and copper, along with a remarkable 727 mg of blood-pressure-lowering potassium.

As mentioned, avocados are unusually high in fat and calories, at least among normally low-calorie fruits and vegetables. That same cup of cubed avocado provides a hearty 240 calories, or about the same amount as in two large bananas, along with 22 grams of fat—about a third of the daily recommendations for an average adult! Yet avocados still come out a winner: 15 of the 22 grams are derived from monounsaturated fat, the key type of fat found in the heart-healthy Mediterranean diet.

AVOCADOS: THE SCIENCE
Avocados, Heart Health, and Weight Control

Perhaps the largest study of the impact of avocados on human health to date was published in early 2013 as part of the National Health and Nutrition Examination Survey (NHANES).[14] This large-scale study, which included more than 17,000 U.S. adults whose dietary habits and health were followed for seven years, examined the potential link between avocado consumption and diet quality, disease risk, and weight control. The results were impressive: Regular avocado consumers tended to eat more fruits and vegetables and had a higher overall quality of diet than their avocado-avoiding counterparts—and this despite a higher average fat intake. Not surprisingly, their intake of dietary fibre, vitamin E, vitamin K, potassium, and magnesium—all

TOP SUPERFOOD SOURCES OF POTASSIUM

FOOD	PORTION	POTASSIUM	POTASSIUM (% DAILY VALUES)
White potato	1 cup, baked in skin (200 g)	1070 mg	31%
Sweet potato	1 cup, baked in skin (200 g)	950 mg	27%
Avocado	1 cup, cubed (150 g)	727 mg	21%
Coconut water	1 cup	600 mg	17%
Kiwi	2 large fruit, without skin (182 g)	568 mg	16%
Lentils	3/4 cup, cooked (149 g)	548 mg	16%
Red kidney beans	3/4 cup, cooked (133 g)	534 mg	15%
Beets	1 cup, cooked (170 g)	518 mg	14%
Black beans	3/4 cup, cooked (129 g)	458 mg	13%
Pomegranate	1 cup arils (174 g)	410 mg	12%
Chickpeas	3/4 cup, cooked (123 g)	357 mg	10%
Amaranth	1 cup, cooked (246 g)	332 mg	9%
Quinoa	1 cup, cooked (185 g)	318 mg	9%
Kale	1 cup, raw (67 g)	299 mg	9%
Pistachios	1 ounce (28 g/49 kernels)	290 mg	8%
Broccoli	1 cup, raw (91 g)	288 mg	8%

Source: USDA National Nutrient Database

nutrients associated with avocados—was higher than in those who avoid them, and they also had higher levels of HDL ("good") cholesterol and a 50% lower risk of metabolic syndrome, the cluster of symptoms associated with type 2 diabetes and heart disease risk, than their peers. But now comes the *pièce de résistance*: Despite the fact that their intake of fat was higher, their total calorie intake was the same as non-eaters, and yet their average weight was actually *lower* than those who eat few to no avocados. Neat.

Although the NHANES results seem compelling, it was a cohort study, and so we don't know if the avocados were causing those effects. To figure out whether or not avocados actually *cause* weight loss (or lower cholesterol or any other measurement), we need controlled clinical trials.

One of the first studies to look directly at the effect of avocados on health was published in 1996 by Mexican researchers, who examined a diet high in monounsaturated fats (MUFAs) from avocados on 30 patients with normal cholesterol and on 37 with high cholesterol or triglycerides (collectively known as lipids).[15] Unfortunately, the study wasn't entirely well designed, but the MUFA-rich diet (which contained the same number of calories as the control diet) did, in fact, bring down total cholesterol in healthy individuals and improved all aspects of the lipid profile (total, HDL, and LDL cholesterol, as well as triglycerides) in those with high cholesterol. Similar results have been found in studies that compared diets with up to three-quarters of daily fat intake from avocados.[16]

Avocados seem to be a healthy choice for people with diabetes, too. In a 1994 study that assigned a group of people with diabetes to follow either a diet high in complex carbohydrates or a diet high in monounsaturated fats, the high-complex-carbohydrate diet brought triglycerides down a little (by 7%) compared with the subjects' usual diet, but the avocado-rich diet brought them down a lot more (20%).[17] Since then, at least five other clinical trials on the effects of avocados have been published, with similar results.[18] Although longer studies are needed, these results strongly suggest that replacing lower-quality carbohydrate foods, such as white bread, white rice, and sweets, with the good fats from avocados could do some real good for our hearts' health.

Avocados and Skin Health

From anti-aging creams to sunscreens to food (avoid sugar, cut back on the booze), the Internet is steeped in suggestions for saving our skin from damage, but how much of it is true? In 2011, a group of researchers from Israel published a study examining the effect of avocado extract on UV damage.[19] When skin cells (keratinocytes) were treated with avocado extract before being exposed to ultraviolet B (UVB) rays, they not only produced fewer inflammatory compounds (known as IL-6 and PGE(2)) but also were better protected from DNA damage. These results, when taken together with an earlier study demonstrating that avocado extracts can improve wound healing in rats,[20] suggest that avocados or avocado extract might play a role in improving or maintaining our skin's health, but, of course, more research in humans is needed.

AVOCADOS: NOT FOR THE BIRDS

Despite all their potential health benefits, avocados aren't for everyone: People with latex allergies can have severe allergic reactions to avocados. Avocado skins and pits are also harmful to many household pets, including dogs, cats, and birds, and are listed as a toxic food for numerous animals by the American Society for the Protection of Cruelty to Animals (ASPCA).[21]

THE BOTTOM LINE

Avocados are amazing, and despite what you might think, they won't cause your waistline to expand if you use them sensibly. Having said that, it bears repeating that if you start eating avocados more often, you're well advised to eat less of something else (think chips and fries). Rich in vitamins, minerals, fibre, and good fats galore, avocados leave little to be desired, both in terms of nutrition and taste. Besides evidence that avocados can help control cholesterol, they may also possess other health effects that are as-yet undiscovered or poorly studied. But I wouldn't advise waiting around for the verdict: When it comes to superfoods, avocados seem to be the real deal.

BEANS, CHICKPEAS, AND LENTILS

The family of foods known as pulses (which includes beans, chickpeas, and lentils) has made virtually every superfood list since the term *superfood* was first coined, but somehow, they still aren't cool. Rich in protein and fibre, pulses are both filling and nutrient dense, not to mention easy on both the pocketbook and the planet.

PULSES: THE STORY

The United Nations' Food and Agriculture Organization defines pulses as the edible dry seeds of leguminous plants. Pulses are differentiated from oil seeds, such as peanuts and other ground nuts, by their low fat content. Among the pulses listed in the FAO's *Codex Alimentarius* are beans of the *Phaseolus* species, such as red, white, and black kidney beans, and the non-*Phaseolus* species, such as lentils, peas, chickpeas, field beans, and cow peas.[22] Beans that are harvested and consumed while still green, including peas and green beans, are classified as vegetables. Although pulses are commonly consumed throughout Central and South America, as well as parts of Africa and Asia, their consumption in the United States, as it is in Canada, remains relatively low, averaging only about 7.5 grams (about 1/4 ounce) per day.[23]

PUTTING PULSES TO USE

Red kidney beans are a natural match for chili, but they are also popular in bean salads, casseroles, soups, dips, and curries as well as pasta fagioli (pasta and bean soup). Black beans can often be interchanged with navy, pinto, or white beans in many recipes and occasionally for red kidney beans. Lentils are available in several varieties, including red and green (the most widely available), along with French Green/Dupuy and Black/Beluga (considered more of a delicacy). Lentils are usually available whole or split; the split lentils tend to be brightly coloured and may look more attractive on your plate, but some of the nutrition is lost when the outer seed coat is removed. On the other hand, split lentils cook more quickly, and the absence of the seed coat makes them better suited for lentil purées. Commonly used in soups and cold bean salads, moderate amounts (usually 1/2 to 1 cup per recipe) of puréed lentils can even be used in baked goods, including brownies, cupcakes, and cookies, where they boost fibre and protein while providing a moist, rich texture. Unlike other beans, lentils do not require soaking before cooking; rinsing and boiling is adequate.

PULSES: THE NUTRITION

In general, pulses are rich in protein, folate, iron, magnesium, potassium, and zinc. They are also exceptionally high in fibre, with most cooked pulses providing between 9 and 12 grams of fibre per 3/4 cup cooked serving. Red kidney beans will also provide you with 14% of

SELECT NUTRIENT CONTENT OF SOME COMMON PULSES

ITEM	Red kidney beans	Black beans	Chickpeas	Lentils
AMOUNT	3/4 cup, cooked (133 g)	3/4 cup, cooked (129 g)	3/4 cup, cooked (123 g)	3/4 cup, cooked (149 g)
Calories	169	170	202	173
Fat	1 g	1 g	3 g	1 g
Carbohydrate	30 g	31 g	34 g	30 g
Fibre	10 g	11 g	9 g	12 g
Protein	11 g	11 g	11 g	13 g
Vitamin B$_1$	14%	21%	10%	17%
Vitamin B$_2$	5%	5%	5%	7%
Vitamin B$_3$	4%	3%	3%	8%
Vitamin B$_6$	8%	5%	8%	14%
Folate	44%	48%	53%	68%
Vitamin K	14%	~	6%	3%
Iron	22%	15%	20%	28%
Magnesium	15%	23%	15%	14%
Potassium	15%	13%	11%	16%
Zinc	10%	10%	13%	13%

Source: USDA National Nutrient Database; - = data not available

your daily vitamin A, while black beans are particularly rich in magnesium and contain anthocyanins, the same compound found in blueberries. Overall, lentils might be the most nutrient dense of the common pulses, with the most protein, fibre, folate, iron, and potassium per 3/4-cup serving.

The deep colour of the red and black beans also implies the presence of antioxidants, and although other foods, especially berries, are richer in total antioxidant content, red kidney and black beans are a particularly rich source of the compound kaempferol, which is not present in white kidney beans. Kaempferol is from a category of plant-based compounds known as flavonoids, which are thought to have active, even medicinal, properties. Found naturally in beans, broccoli, tea, kale, and strawberries, a high intake of kaempferol has been associated with a lower risk of some types of cancer as well as heart disease.[24] Unfortunately, while kaempferol from beans is quite readily absorbed by the human body, the downside is that it inhibits the absorption of iron from the bean.[25] White kidney beans, by comparison, contain no kaempferol or other flavonoids, which means the bioavailability of the iron is higher, making them a more suitable choice for those with, or at risk for, iron deficiency.[26]

PULSES: THE SCIENCE

Unfortunately, compared with other superfoods, such as almonds or green tea, there is a relative dearth of research on pulses as a whole, and the research on individual pulses, such as lentils, is scarce. We do know, however, that individuals who eat more pulses tend to do a better job meeting their overall nutrient needs: According to an analysis of the 2004 Canadian Community Health Survey, regular pulse consumers had higher intakes of fibre, folate, potassium, phosphorus, magnesium, iron, and zinc than those who rarely, or never, consume beans, chickpeas, and lentils.[27]

WHAT IS A COHORT STUDY?

Population studies examine the association between foods or lifestyle choices and health-related outcomes, such as obesity, type 2 diabetes, heart disease, or even death (all-cause mortality) in a large group of individuals, or cohort, for years or even decades. These cohort studies are helpful for finding associations between habits, behaviours, or exposures (for example, smoking, sunshine, or pollutants) and the outcomes related to health or disease. The results of cohort studies often serve as a catalyst for more research to understand more precisely why the relationship might exist. Notably, population studies suggest a correlation, or connection, between the exposure and the outcome; they do not prove that one causes the other. In other words, just because one habit or behaviour is found to be associated with a higher or lower risk of disease in a cohort study doesn't mean it was the cause; there could be a separate but related cause that is associated with both, or the relationship could be mere coincidence. For example, low vitamin D status is associated with heart disease risk, but it is not yet clear whether or not vitamin D actually prevents heart disease, or if it is just a marker for other factors associated with it. People with higher vitamin D status, for example, tend to be outside in the sun more often, being active and living a healthier lifestyle, and that could be the real reason why people with higher vitamin D status seem to have healthier hearts.

Pulses and Overall Disease Risk

Cohort studies have demonstrated that bean consumption is associated with a reduced risk of disease, including type 2 diabetes. An Australian study examining dietary factors associated with mortality (death rates) in long-lived elderly people in Japan, Sweden, Greece, and Australia found that, for every 20 grams of legumes (pulses) consumed per day, mortality risk dropped by 7% to 8% over a five-year period (1/2 cup of beans is about 90 grams, so 20 grams is a pretty small portion).[28]

A larger study, part of the well-documented National Health and Nutrition Examination Survey (NHANES) Epidemiologic Follow-Up Study, examined the association between legume intake and cardiovascular disease (CVD) risk. After 19 years of follow-up in a group of nearly 10,000 men and women, those who ate legumes at least four times per week were at a 22% lower risk of coronary heart disease and an 11% lower risk of cardiovascular disease versus those who consumed legumes less than once per week.[29] In a study of a subset of participants with diabetes in the large-scale European Prospective Investigation into Cancer and Nutrition (EPIC) study, intake of fruit, vegetables, and legumes together was associated with a reduced risk of all-cause mortality, meaning dying of any cause, as well as risk of death from cardiovascular disease. When the three categories of food were analyzed separately, however, the trend toward reduced risk of all-cause mortality was true only for vegetables and legumes, not fruit.[30] Of course, although these studies don't prove causation, they certainly provide fodder to consider putting a few meatless meals on the menu.

Part of the benefit of beans on CVD risk could be related to their soluble, viscous fibre content, which can support healthy cholesterol control. In a study conducted by researchers at the University of Saskatchewan and published in the *British Journal of Nutrition*, 108 older adults (aged 50 and over) were given two servings, or about 150 grams (dry weight), of beans, chickpeas, peas, or lentils per day for two months and assessed for CVD risk factors compared with their regular diets. After two months on the pulse-based diet, the subjects saw their total cholesterol drop by 8.3% and their LDL cholesterol by 7.9%.[31]

Pulses also tend to support healthy blood sugar control in people with and without diabetes. Beans and lentils can help reduce the glycemic (blood sugar) effect of a meal, which is not surprising when you consider their glycemic index: Lentils, for example, have an amazingly low GI of 31 (any GI under 55 is considered low).[32,33]

BEAN POISONING?

Perhaps the most concerning side effect associated with eating beans is the potential for phytohemagglutinin poisoning in uncooked and undercooked beans, especially red kidney beans. Phytohemagglutinin (PHA) is a lectin, a type of protein found naturally in plant and some animal foods, that can become toxic to humans at high levels and possibly make food allergies to beans more severe.[34] Although lectins are present in all beans, PHA is most concentrated in red kidney beans. PHA poisoning, which is associated with severe and short-lived nausea, vomiting, and diarrhea that sets in as little as three hours after consumption, can be caused by as few as four or five uncooked beans. Fortunately, the toxins can be deactivated by boiling the beans for as little as 10 minutes.[35] In that time, the number of toxins drops from 20,000 to 70,000 hemagglutinating units, or hau, in raw red kidney beans to 200 to 400 hau in cooked beans (note that white kidney beans have about one-third the PHA content of red beans). Importantly, the beans must be in boiling (100°C) water: PHA poisoning has been reported in beans cooked at lower temperatures, such as in slow cookers, where the temperature may not exceed 75 to 80°C.

Although PHA toxins can be deactivated in as little as 10 minutes, the U.S. Food and Drug Administration recommends a 30-minute boil to ensure the beans have reached a sufficient temperature to destroy all the lectin (note that canned beans are precooked). You can use canned beans for added safety (if you're concerned about bisphenol A, or BPA, a plastic-derived substance that has been banned from baby bottles but still exists in the lining of cans, try companies such as Eden Organic, which sell their beans in BPA-free cans). If you soak your beans overnight, make sure to discard the water (this is key!) before boiling.

CONSEQUENCES OF CONSUMPTION

Pulses, such as kidney beans, are of particular importance for developing nations. Rich in energy and providing two to three times more protein than many cereal grains, pulses also tend to be good sources of iron and calcium, although the bioavailability (ability of the human body to access the nutrients) varies from pulse to pulse. As of 2001, developing countries consumed an estimated 90% of the pulses grown for humans, contributing about 10% of the protein and 5% of the calories consumed in lower-income countries.[36]

Pulses also have good potential to help our struggling environment. One of the key steps in the process of formulating fertilizers is nitrogen fixation, an energy-intensive process that usually requires input from petroleum products. Ironically, nitrogen fixation is so energy-intensive that the energy that goes into producing the fertilizer often exceeds the output of energy in the crop that is actually produced.[37] (This is why many environmentalists are concerned about biofuels, which are often produced from corn, a crop that is significantly fertilizer-dependent.) When it comes to the environment, then, lentils and other pulses are true superfoods: They are a rare crop that actually fixes nitrogen, naturally adding it back to the soil. For that reason, they are often used as part of a crop rotation with wheat. Lentils also grow well in cool, dry conditions and are relatively stable during drought.

THE BOTTOM LINE

Whether it's lentils, chickpeas, or beans, any kind of pulse can make a sensible addition to many diets. With research suggesting they may contribute to cholesterol control, and with a possible protective effect against diabetes, pulses are nutritious and might be worth a bit more of our collective attention.

BEETS

If you're not a fan of borscht, there is a reasonable chance that beets don't make their way onto your dinner plate. Even as recently as a few years ago, beets didn't have a lot of bragging rights, except, of course, for being able to make great stains on white clothing. All of that changed around 2006, when the first studies on the role of beetroot juice (the juice of the beet) on exercise performance were published. It didn't take long for sports science enthusiasts to latch onto the data, and before we knew it, beets became a big deal.

BEETS: THE STORY

Beets are the root of the *Beta vulgaris* plant, which is a member of the goosefoot, or Chenopodiaceae, family. Beets exist in four forms: (1) the garden beet, or beetroot—that's the beet you'll see in the grocery store or at a farmers' market; (2) the sugar beet, which is used for sugar production; (3) the mangel-wurzel, or mangold, which is used for livestock; and (4) the leaf beet, or Swiss chard, itself a familiar name in the world of superfoods.[38] The garden beet, or beetroot, comes in several colours, including deep magenta, yellow, and even candy cane (striped).

BEETS: THE NUTRITION

Despite their deep red appearance, beets are decent, but not outstanding, in terms of their basic vitamin and mineral content: A cup (170 grams) of boiled beets provides 74 calories, 3 grams of fibre, and

3 grams of protein. The 34% of your folate they provide is comparable to green vegetables and beans and pulses. They also kick in a healthy 14% (518 mg) of your potassium, an amount that exceeds bananas, and serve as a source of vitamin C (10%), iron (8%), copper (6%), and vitamin B$_6$ (6%). That's nothing to be ashamed of, but it's not record-breaking, either.

BEETS: THE SCIENCE
Beets and Blood Pressure

This is where it gets interesting. The recent affection for beets centres not on their vitamin or mineral content but on their nitrate content. Yes, that's nitrate, as in the stuff in bacon and bologna that we associate with cancer risk. The story centres around a compound known as nitric oxide, or NO, which acts on the walls of our arteries (called the endothelium) to relax them. Relaxed, or vasodilated, arteries allow better blood flow, which should not only reduce blood pressure but also improve the health of our entire vascular system. On the other hand, as we gain weight, especially around the middle, or when we smoke, don't eat properly, or don't exercise, our NO levels tend to drop, and our arteries become more constricted. Men with erectile dysfunction tend to have low circulating levels of NO, and it is believed that the same dietary and lifestyle habits that trigger heart disease—along with the associated low levels of NO—can trigger erectile dysfunction (and vice versa; adopting a Mediterranean-style diet seems to reverse erectile dysfunction).[39]

As it turns out, eating nitrate-rich foods—of which beets are one of the richest—has a positive effect on the body's NO levels. Since NO relaxes our arteries, researchers have turned their attention to the effect of nitrates on blood pressure, and the effect appears to be significant: In a combined 16 studies, including 254 total participants, taking beetroot juice or an equivalent nitrate-containing supplement brought down systolic blood pressure (that's the top number) by 4.4 mm Hg and diastolic blood pressure (the bottom number) by 1.1 mg Hg.[40] By comparison, cutting your salt intake—an onerous task for many—can reduce systolic blood pressure only slightly more, by about 7 mm Hg.[41]

EATING BEETS

Believe it or not, beets are really easy to prepare. If you can cook a potato, then you can cook a beet—and if you can't cook a potato, then that's another matter. Here are the basics:

Take your beets by the roots, cut off the greens (which you can prepare in the same way as any other dark, leafy green), and boil them with the skins on (this will help retain the moisture) until they are soft like a boiled potato. Remove from the water, and take the peel off with a knife or your fingers once they have cooled a little. Cut into medallions or small cubes, toss with a bit of olive oil, pepper, and a touch of salt, if desired, and that's it—they are ready to serve.

Alternatively, you can toss the cooked beets with olive oil, parmesan cheese, and balsamic vinegar and serve them warm. Or cool them and serve as a salad with a bit of sour cream and fresh dill. If you want an even simpler and lower-calorie method of preparing beets, however, just wrap them in foil and put them on the barbecue until they are tender—you don't even need salt or oil.

Beets and Athletic Performance

Now, back to the story about beets and athletic performance. The production of NO was long thought to take place only one way: via the conversion of the amino acid L-arginine to L-citrulline (don't worry, you don't need to memorize this). Since this process needs plenty of oxygen to be completed, it didn't make much sense that manipulating NO would improve your workout, since oxygen is in relatively short supply when our muscles are hard at work. That is, until a second path, in which NO is produced from the nitrates we eat in food—and which can occur even when oxygen is in short supply—was discovered in the mid-1990s.[42]

In this second pathway, naturally occurring nitrate (scientifically denoted as NO_3) from food is converted into nitrite (NO_2)—note the spelling—by bacteria in our mouths. Nitrite is then converted to NO in our stomachs and beyond, and off it goes to do its job. Interestingly, using mouthwash abolishes this process because it kills the good bacteria in our mouths that help convert NO_3 to NO_2. So much for fresh breath. As mentioned, this entire process can occur when oxygen is in short supply, as would be the case during exercise. So, by eating nitrate-rich foods, such as beets or beetroot juice, it's believed you can increase blood flow to your muscles, helping them work more efficiently, especially during intense exercise. And while fruits and vegetables provide about 60% to 80% of the nitrate we eat (note that nitrate from vegetables does not appear to be associated with cancer risk, as may be the case with cured and preserved meats),[43] beets are one of the richest sources around.

Now, that's a nice theory, but what about the evidence? It turns out that a number of studies have, in fact, demonstrated that beetroot juice can help improve sport performance by about 2%, a small but significant edge, especially in competitive situations.[44] A recent trial published in the *Journal of the Academy of Nutrition and Dietetics* found that runners who ate about a half pound of cooked beets two hours before a run ran faster over 5 km than those who didn't; and yet, their heart rates were the same.[45] Perhaps most important for the majority of the population who aren't winning Olympic medals, the benefits of beets and other nitrate-rich foods seem to be most pronounced in weekend warriors and recreational athletes—basically, non-elite athletes.[46] In other words, beets might help the average person work out at a higher intensity, which could help less-serious exercisers enjoy the experience more.

BEET PEE?

No doubt, the biggest side effect associated with beets (other than unexplained bursts of speed) is something known as beeturia, namely somewhat red-hued pee or poop that many experience after eating beets. Although utterly alarming at first, if you ate beets before you saw the red in the toilet bowl, don't panic, as it will go away on its own. On the other hand, if you experience blood in your stool (or urine) any other time, then it's definitely worth a trip to the doctor's office to get to the bottom of the situation.

THE BOTTOM LINE

Who could have imagined that an unassuming red root could not only be healthy but could actually help us run faster, too—and feel better while we're at it? Perhaps even more important, the emerging research on beets and beetroot juice has ignited a whole new debate on the role that dietary nitrates—at least the ones not associated with cold cuts—could play in our health. As we unravel the intriguing story of how NO works in our bodies, it becomes increasingly clear that beets (and spinach and other nitrate-rich foods) could play a vital role in the health of our entire vascular system, making them a superfood in the truest sense.

BLUEBERRIES

For years, both cultivated and wild blueberries have enjoyed the proud image of being a source of antioxidants and a natural defense against aging. But digging a bit below the surface reveals the reality that the blueberry story is a bit more complex than many of the health magazines will tell you.

BLUEBERRIES: THE STORY

Blueberries largely exist in two forms: wild (*Vaccinium angustifolium*) and cultivated, of which there are numerous varieties. Both types of blueberries are part of the Ericaceae, or heather, family, which is botanically distinct from strawberries, raspberries, and blackberries. Wild blueberries, also known as lowbush berries, are a relatively special find, with a growing region that includes only Canada and parts of Maine. Unlike cultivated, or highbush, blueberries, which are planted, wild blueberries are pollinated by bees and spread underground by rhizomes, in much the same way that mushrooms spread. Wild blueberries are one of only three berries native to North America and have reportedly been consumed by aboriginal populations for at least 10,000 years. They were first harvested commercially in the Civil War, where they helped feed the Union Army, but now they feed an army of health-conscious citizens as a hot-ticket item in midsummer farmers' markets.

No doubt, Canadians have a close relationship with our native berry. Annual consumption has nearly quadrupled since the early 1980s, with the average Canadian eating about 0.8 kg (800 grams) of blueberries per year, an amount that exceeds all other berries, other than strawberries, combined.[47] Blueberries are big business for Canadian fruit farmers, making up about 16% of all fruit-farm cash receipts in 2009, an amount that trailed only apples and grapes. Canadian blueberries are also in hot demand around the world and make up one of Canada's top fruit exports.

BLUEBERRIES: THE NUTRITION

Cultivated blueberries are naturally low in calories, providing just 84 calories' worth of energy per 1-cup (148 gram) serving, along with 4 grams of fibre. It might surprise you, however, to know that aside from their fibre content, cultivated blueberries are an excellent source of only a handful of vitamins and minerals: A cup will provide you with a quarter of your day's vitamin C, a third of your vitamin K, and a quarter of your manganese needs, a mineral that is prevalent in a wide array of foods. Otherwise, they don't provide more than 4% of your daily requirement of any other single nutrient, along with no significant amount of protein or healthy fats.

But what about wild blueberries? They are purported to be more nutrient dense than cultivated blueberries; where do they stack up? A cup of wild blueberries is slightly lower in calories than their cultivated cousins (71 in wild vs. 84 in cultivated) and provide 50% more fibre (6 vs. 4 grams). On the other hand, cultivated blueberries provide more vitamins B_1, B_2, C, E, and folate than their wild cousins.

So, why all the fuss? Much of the attention afforded to blueberries, and other berries, is derived from their antioxidant content. A landmark study published in the *American Journal of Clinical Nutrition* in 2006, for example, found that blueberries ranked among the top 10 foods for antioxidant content per serving size (notably, 5 of the top 10 foods were berries),[48] and wild blueberries are richer than cultivated blueberries. Among beverages, blueberry juice has been ranked behind only pomegranate juice, red wine, and concord grape

KEY NUTRIENTS FOUND IN FOUR COMMON NORTH AMERICAN BERRIES

ITEM	Blueberries, cultivated	Blueberries, wild	Strawberries	Rasp -berries	Black -berries
AMOUNT	1 cup, raw (148 g)	1 cup, raw (140 g)	1 cup, halves (152 g)	1 cup, raw (123 g)	1 cup, raw (144 g)
Calories	84	71	49	64	62
Fat	0 g	0 g	0 g	1 g	1 g
Carbohydrate	21 g	18 g	12 g	15 g	15 g
Fibre	4 g	6 g	3 g	8 g	8 g
Protein	1 g	0 g	1 g	1 g	2 g
Vitamin B_1	4%	2%	2%	3%	2%
Vitamin B_2	4%	0%	2%	3%	2%
Vitamin B_3	3%	4%	3%	4%	5%
Vitamin B_6	4%	2%	4%	3%	2%
Folate	2%	~	9%	6%	9%
Vitamin C	24%	4%	149%	54%	50%
Vitamin K	36%	~	4%	12%	36%
Iron	2%	4%	3%	5%	5%
Magnesium	2%	2%	5%	7%	7%
Potassium	2%	3%	7%	5%	7%
Zinc	2%	8%	1%	3%	5%

Source: USDA National Nutrient Database (all except wild blueberries, retrieved from www. wildblueberries.com/health/nutrition-facts.php); - = data not available

juice for its antioxidant capacity.[49] Unfortunately, the link between antioxidants and health outcomes has come into question, leaving us to wonder whether these bragging rights are meaningful or not.

BLUEBERRIES: THE SCIENCE
Although there has been a significant amount of research on the effect

of blueberries on cognitive function (including memory and decision making), heart disease, and cancer risk, there are actually very few well-controlled human studies that have either directly compared blueberries with a placebo or have used blueberries as part of a dietary intervention program, as has been the case with almonds and strawberries. But, for what it's worth, here is some of the data we have available today.

Blueberries and Heart Health

A number of observational studies—the types of studies that involve monitoring the habits or food choices of a large group of individuals, then correlating them to disease risk—have demonstrated that blueberries and other foods rich in anthocyanins, a plant compound that helps give blueberries their distinctive colour, may have positive effects on human health. The most recent, published in 2013, included nearly 100,000 women who have been followed since 1989 as part of the Nurses' Health Study; it found that the women who had the highest intake of anthocyanins had the lowest risk of heart attack.[50]

Since cohort studies can suggest only correlation, not causation, we need to look to randomized controlled trials to see whether or not blueberries actually can protect our hearts. To date, only one randomized trial, published in the *Journal of Nutrition* in 2010, has examined the effect of blueberry consumption on cardiovascular risk factors.[51] In this particular study, 48 obese men and women with metabolic syndrome (the cluster of symptoms associated with an increased risk of developing type 2 diabetes and heart disease) and prehypertension (borderline high blood pressure) were given either a freeze-dried blueberry drink, equivalent to about 2 cups of blueberries, or an equal amount of water, every day for eight weeks.

At the end of the study, those who downed the blueberry drink saw their blood pressure drop significantly (their systolic blood pressure, the top number, dropped by 6%, while their diastolic blood pressure, the bottom number, dropped by 4%) compared with those who stuck to water. Less impressive were the results from their blood sugar control and cholesterol profile, as well as measures of inflammation (including the compound C-reactive protein), all of which were unchanged. In the blueberries' favour, the researchers did find a drop in oxidative damage to LDL ("bad") cholesterol (oxidation of LDL cholesterol is believed to be one of the triggers of plaque buildup that can precipitate heart attacks and strokes) in the blueberry group versus controls. The fact that the participants had normal LDL cholesterol and blood sugar levels to begin with, however, could explain why the blueberries seemingly had little effect on their collective risk factors: It's possible their effect is more potent on individuals who are already at risk.

Blueberries and the Brain

Animal studies suggesting that blueberries play a role in brain function, possibly delaying cognitive decline and slowing the onset of Alzheimer's disease, have received their fair share of attention. As for human studies, the same Nurses' Health Study found that cognitive decline began 1.5 to 2.5 years later for those who consumed the most blueberries and strawberries versus those who consumed the least.[52] In clinical trials, only one small study, conducted jointly by researchers at the University of Cincinnati, Agriculture and Agri-Food Canada, and the USDA Human Nutrition Research Center on Aging, and funded by the Wild Blueberry Association of North America, has been conducted.[53] The study found that daily intake of wild blueberry juice improved learning and recall over a 12-week period in a small group of older adults with early memory changes. The study was a preliminary one, however, and as result did not include a control group. Although these studies suggest that blueberries might have some type of effect on brain health, especially as we age, the data on humans is remarkably thin.

Blueberries and Oxidative Stress

Oxidative stress is thought to be a contributing factor to aging and a number of health-related issues, including heart disease and possibly cancer risk. A 2002 study found that taking freeze-dried blueberry powder with a meal resulted in a significant increase in circulating antioxidant levels in the bloodstreams of a group of middle-aged men, but the study was small and did not link the increased antioxidant status with any health outcomes or disease risk factors.[54] A more recent study found that runners who ate 250 grams of blueberries per day (that's about a half pound) for six weeks had higher levels of natural killer (NK) cells, cells whose job it is to put older or damaged cells out of their misery.[55] They also found that a pre-exercise dose of blueberries (375 grams taken an hour before two and a half hours of running) reduced markers of inflammation and oxidative stress that are often associated with high-intensity physical activity. To date, however, no study has provided a clear link between blueberry consumption and disease outcomes that could be related to oxidative stress.

Blueberries and Blood Sugar Control

A number of studies have suggested that blueberries, and other berries, can improve blood sugar control. Unfortunately, since the majority of these studies have been in animals or cell lines, the relationship in humans is less certain. This issue was at least partially addressed by British researchers, who found in 2011 that adding blueberries or raspberries to pancakes didn't do anything to reduce the blood sugar effect of pancakes made with plain glucose or fructose.[56] On the other hand, a randomized, double-blind, placebo-controlled trial on obese men and women with insulin resistance (prediabetes) found that those who drank a daily smoothie containing bioactive compounds derived from blueberries improved their insulin sensitivity after six weeks, versus a control group who consumed the daily smoothie without the blueberry supplement.[57] This would suggest that blueberries may have some effect on long-term blood sugar control (versus immediate effects in the pancake study), but once again, the effect seems to be most pronounced in those who are already at an increased risk of developing disease.

THE BOTTOM LINE

Blueberries may well be one of the original superfoods, but the truth is, we really don't have as much hard data on their ability to ward off disease in humans as we might have assumed. Of course, the question of wild versus cultivated berries always looms large; since most of the available research is on the cultivated variety, it is possible that wild blueberries may have more of an effect on disease risk than their cultivated cousins. Nonetheless, blueberries should still be welcome in almost any diet, not only for their fibre, vitamin C, and vitamin K content but also for their great taste, which makes it easy for many of us to enjoy getting our daily fruit.

BROCCOLI

When in Doubt, Eat Broccoli[58] is the title of dietitian Liz Pearson's 1998 book on the now-ubiquitous green veggie. Although broccoli might have been one of the first popularized North American superfoods, with so much competition nowadays, it feels almost a bit milquetoast. So, where does broccoli actually stand in an increasingly crowded world of supervegetables?

BROCCOLI: THE STORY

A member of the same *Brassica*, or mustard (Brassicaceae) family as cauliflower, cabbage, and Brussels sprouts, broccoli (*Brassica oleracea*, variety *italica*) made its way into our collective consciousness as a potential cure-all for cancer prevention, heart disease, and aging. Its history, however, is much longer, dating back to ancient Rome, where it was first cultivated, eventually making its way to England in the early 1700s, where it likely thrived in the cooler climate. It is said that early use of broccoli in the United States can be traced back to Italian immigrants who brought it to New York City.[59]

The *B. oleracea* species includes a wide range of vegetables we commonly consume today, ranging from broccoli to kale to kohlrabi, but you'll also find other familiar foods in the wider *Brassica* family, including rutabaga and turnip. Amazingly, despite all the hype, broccoli was, as of 2010, only the 11th-most-consumed vegetable by Canadians, behind the likes of lettuce, onions, cucumbers, pumpkins and squash, and of course, potatoes.[60]

BROCCOLI: THE NUTRITION

As with all non-starchy vegetables, broccoli is low in calories: A cup of chopped raw broccoli provides a modest 31 calories' worth of energy, along with 2.4 grams of fibre. Perhaps most impressive, however, a cup of broccoli is a top food source of vitamin C, providing 135% of your daily requirements—more than a medium orange—along with more than a day's worth of bone-building vitamin K (116%).

Although vitamin C and vitamin K are broccoli's headline nutrients, it also provides 11% of your vitamin A (as the plant form, beta-carotene) and 14% of your folate, as well as 288 mg, or 8%, of your daily potassium requirements. Broccoli also contains lutein, a nutrient thought to be important for protecting our eyes as we age.[61]

Like kale, broccoli is a relatively uncommon green vegetable that is low in oxalates, the compounds that bind calcium and cause it to be lost in your urine. High-oxalate foods, which include Swiss chard and spinach, can possibly increase your risk of kidney stones if consumed in very large amounts, so broccoli eaters are doubly lucky.

BROCCOLI: THE SCIENCE

Although studies specifically examining the role of broccoli on human health do exist, most studies have examined the role of cruciferous vegetables (vegetables from the *Brassica* family) as a whole, with perhaps the most powerful data relating to their possible role in cancer prevention. For example, there is some evidence, albeit not always consistent, that cruciferous vegetables protect against colorectal cancer: The most recent meta-analysis, or study that pools results from previous trials, found that those who consumed the most cruciferous vegetables had an 18% lower risk of developing colorectal cancer versus those who ate the least.[62] A 2011 study in the *International Journal of Cancer* also found that, for every 25 grams of *Brassica* vegetables eaten per day (you'll get about three times that much in 1/2 cup of cooked, chopped broccoli), the risk of developing a type of stomach cancer, known as gastric cardia adenocarcinoma, dropped by 28%.[63] Other studies have demonstrated that a higher consumption of green vegetables is associated not only with better blood sugar control in people with type 2 diabetes but also a lower body weight and reduced triglycerides.[64]

But what about broccoli, specifically? Unfortunately, it's virtually impossible to create a true double-blind, placebo-controlled trial, the true gold standard of clinical research, on a food such as broccoli. The entire premise of these controlled trials is to have one group take a dummy pill (the placebo, or control, group) while the other takes the food or supplement you wish to study (the intervention group). In the best studies, the subjects don't know what they are taking and the researchers don't know, either—that's the nature of the process known as "blinding." Blinding is used to make sure the subjects aren't influenced by the placebo effect, but it's also important for the researchers to be blinded, to prevent conscious or unconscious bias from leaking into a study. For example, if researchers are aware of who is getting the treatment food, supplement, or drug, they may treat that group differently from the control group, which can have an effect on the outcome of the study.

But how can you hide the fact that you're giving one group broccoli and the other group nothing? That's not exactly easy. Yes, you could purée the broccoli and hide it in other foods, such as a smoothie, but if the taste, appearance, or texture of the smoothie differs from what the controls are receiving, then the study isn't exactly blind anymore. For this reason, it's common to use dried, powdered forms of some fruits or vegetables, which can then be taken just like any pill, including the placebo. The plus side is you get a better-controlled study, particularly as it relates to the active compounds in the food; the downside, however, is that you don't necessarily have as realistic a picture of what happens when you eat the food in its most natural form.

Nonetheless, studies using powdered fruits or vegetables are at times the best we can do, and in the case of broccoli, a number of studies have used broccoli sprouts powder (BSP) to give a better idea of what broccoli may have to offer. A recent study examining the impact of BSP on people with type 2 diabetes, for example, found that four weeks of consuming 10 grams per day of BSP (equivalent to about 1 cup of fresh broccoli) resulted in less oxidation of LDL cholesterol and higher levels of antioxidants in the bloodstream.[65] As a reminder, when LDL, or the so-called bad cholesterol, is oxidized, it is effectively damaged, a process that is thought to be an early step in the development of plaques in our arteries. By preventing oxidative damage to LDL cholesterol, then, broccoli—at least in its powdered form—may help keep the hearts of people with type 2 diabetes, and anyone else at risk of CVD, healthy. Unfortunately, although some studies have demonstrated the benefits of BSP, others have not. For example, a similar four-week study demonstrated no benefits of taking 10 grams per day of BSP on blood pressure and related measures.[66]

BITTER BROCCOLI?

No doubt the biggest obstacle to getting people—especially kids—to eat broccoli is its slightly bitter taste, which is attributed to the sulfur-containing compound 6-n-propylthiouracil. If you've never noticed this distinctive taste and smell, however, it's probably not your imagination: Our genes dictate whether we find 6-n-propylthiouracil bitter or not. So, what to do if you, or your kids, are on the unlucky side of the bitter gene? Pass the dressing: A study by researchers at Temple University found that offering dip improved the consumption of broccoli among preschoolers who were genetically sensitive to bitterness (interestingly, those who weren't genetically sensitive to bitterness ate the same amount of broccoli, regardless of whether or not dip was served).[67] And while the calorie-conscious might cringe at the notion of ratcheting up low-calorie veggies with fat-laden dips, there might be good reason to do so: According to Japanese researchers, levels of lutein and zeaxanthin, nutrients found in broccoli that are thought to be important for eye health, as well as beta-carotene, were highest in the bloodstreams of subjects who ate broccoli with mayonnaise—yes, mayonnaise—versus those who ate broccoli plain or even with oil.[68]

THE BOTTOM LINE

It might not feel as cool and new-agey as it did a decade ago, but broccoli is still a sure bet. Nutrient dense and backed by a decent body of research, along with the rest of its cruciferous cousins, broccoli is an old-school superfood that shouldn't be forgotten in the new world of healthy eating.

GREEN TEA

If you pick up just about any weight-loss supplement on the market today, odds are pretty good you'll find an ingredient called EGCG on the list. The popular fat-burner is derived from green tea, and if you believe the hype, green tea or its extract will get you lean and mean in no time and keep you cancer-free for life.

GREEN TEA: THE STORY

Green tea is a traditional drink in Asia. Thanks in part to research suggesting it confers a number of possible health benefits, its popularity has increased the world over. Derived from the *Camellia sinensis* plant, green tea is not fermented, setting it apart from oolong tea, which is partly fermented, and black tea, which is fully fermented. Interestingly, the more a tea is fermented, the lower its content of potentially disease-fighting polyphenols and the higher its caffeine content.

GREEN TEA: THE NUTRITION

Since green tea, like coffee, black tea, and herbal teas, is a calorie-free beverage (or close enough), it is also not a source of protein, carbohydrates, fats, or fibre. Its vitamin and mineral content is also insignificant. So, why the perceived magical powers? It seems to stem from the polyphenols, and in particular, a group of flavonols (a type of polyphenol) known as catechins, that are found in green tea. Over the years, research has focused on the effects of green tea as a beverage and on the catechins as supplements. Of the six catechins found in green tea, the most potent appears to be epigallocatechin gallate, or EGCG, so it's no surprise it is also the best studied.

Like black tea and coffee, green tea does contain caffeine as well as other stimulating compounds, including theobromine and theophylline, albeit in smaller amounts: A typical 8-ounce (250 ml) cup of brewed green tea provides about 30 mg of caffeine, about two-thirds of the amount in black tea.[69]

High doses of green tea also supply significant amounts of oxalates, compounds associated with certain types of kidney stones, though the real (versus perceived) impact of oxalates in the diet on kidney stones is a matter of some debate.[70] Compounds in green tea are also thought to bind to iron, especially from plant foods, increasing the risk of iron deficiency, which is particularly common in children and women of child-bearing age. Although drinking tea doesn't seem to be an issue for the iron status of healthy individuals, it could be a problem if your iron status is already low.[71]

GREEN TEA: THE SCIENCE

Green tea is easily one of the most-researched foods or beverages of any kind. In fact, it is so well studied that researchers have been able to compile several meta-analyses (compilations of data from previous studies to create a better statistical picture of its effects), including the *Cochrane Database of Systematic Reviews,* the gold standard for independent critical evaluation of evidence.

Green Tea and Weight Loss

Numerous studies have suggested that green tea might actually have some kind of an effect on our weight, possibly because of those catechins, or possibly because of its caffeine content, or maybe a bit of both. Either way, it's thought that green tea increases something known as thermogenesis, or the number of calories your body burns, after you drink it. In December 2012, a *Cochrane Review* on the effect of green tea on weight loss put this theory to the test, by compiling all the available data from studies that have been done on overweight and obese individuals (that's an important detail: This was not a compilation of data on gym-goers looking to lose the last 5 pounds).[72] To make sure they were using only the best studies, the authors included only randomized controlled trials (considered the best, least-biased form of research) that were at least 3 months long. All told, only six studies were deemed to be of high enough quality to meet the criteria. Among the included studies, involving a total of 532 participants, the average weight loss was (drum roll, please) 0.04 kg. Not into metric? That's 0.09 pounds. Ouch.

But wait! What if green tea targets weight in one particular part of the body, such as belly fat, more than anywhere else? The *Cochrane Review* team looked at that as well. They assessed the impact of green tea on waist circumference, an indicator of visceral fat, the deep fat around your organs that is associated with an increased risk of type 2 diabetes, heart disease, and cancer. Once again, the results were as skinny as the jeans you'd imagine yourself wearing if you drank enough of the green stuff: The five studies included in the analysis saw a whopping 0.2 cm drop off the midsections of 404 subjects— yes, that's an average of 2 *millimeters* off their waistlines. The bottom line? The *Cochrane Review* team found that "green tea preparations appear to induce a small, statistically non-significant weight loss in overweight and obese adults. Because the amount of weight loss is small, it is not likely to be clinically important."

Green Tea and Cardiovascular Health

While green tea might be a dud when it comes to weight loss, the notion that it could protect against heart disease emerged from studies suggesting that individuals who drank more than two cups of green tea per day had lower levels of total cholesterol and were at a remarkable 22% to 33% lower risk of dying from heart disease than their peers.[73,74] More recently, a meta-analysis suggested that, for every one-cup increase in green tea consumption, the risk of coronary artery disease (another way of saying heart disease) declines by an impressive 10%.[75]

Just how could green tea protect the heart? Early animal studies suggested it might prevent absorption of cholesterol by the digestive system while also increasing the expression of proteins that remove LDL ("bad") cholesterol from the bloodstream. In 2011, the first two meta-analyses on the effects of green tea or green tea extract on lipid (meaning cholesterol and triglyceride) levels in humans were published, just months apart. In the first, published by Chinese research- ers in the *American Journal of Clinical Nutrition* in August 2011, a total of 14 studies were pooled.[76] The studies were at least two weeks long, using green tea or green tea extract while keeping diets otherwise unchanged (this is important to make sure the effect is from green tea, and not due to weight loss or other dietary changes). In total, the researchers found that green tea reduced total cholesterol by 0.19 mmol/L and LDL cholesterol by 0.06 mmol/L. The second study combined a total of 20 randomized controlled trials and found a similar drop in total cholesterol and LDL cholesterol of 0.14 mmol/L compared with controls.[77]

Although these results seem to suggest green tea can help lower cholesterol, the effects are small; most people's total cholesterol is in the range of 4 to 6 mmol/L (anything above 5.2 mmol/L is considered high), with an LDL of between 2.0 and 5.0 mmol/L. In other words, a drop of 0.1 mmol/L or so isn't going to keep many people off medication. On the other hand, the quality of the studies used in these meta-analyses was mixed; only a handful of studies were considered to be of the highest quality, and the doses of green tea catechins varied considerably, making it difficult to determine just how effective green tea really is and whether or not a higher dose could offer more benefit. Finally, there is a possible confounding effect of caffeine: Research on coffee suggests that caffeine might increase total cholesterol,[78] and since green tea is mildly caffeinated, that could drag cholesterol numbers upward. Perhaps decaf green tea is the best choice?

Green Tea and Blood Sugar

In a 2013 meta-analysis that included 22 studies and more than 1,500 subjects, green tea or green tea supplements brought fasting blood sugars down by 0.08 mmol/L over 12 weeks; by comparison, an average person's blood sugar is around 5 mmol/L, while diabetes can be diagnosed once fasting sugars consistently exceed 6 mmol/L.[79] In other words, the effect of green tea on blood sugar appears to be

CAFFEINE CONTENT OF SOME COMMON FOODS AND DRINKS

PRODUCT	SERVING SIZE	CAFFEINE CONTENT
Coffee, brewed	1 cup/8 ounces/237 ml	135 mg
Coffee, roasted and ground, percolated	1 cup/8 ounces/237 ml	118 mg
Coffee, roasted and ground, filter drip	1 cup/8 ounces/237 ml	179 mg
Coffee, roasted and ground, decaffeinated	1 cup/8 ounces/237 ml	3 mg
Coffee, instant	1 cup/8 ounces/237 ml	76–106 mg
Tea, average blend	1 cup/8 ounces/237 ml	43 mg
Tea, green	1 cup/8 ounces/237 ml	30 mg
Tea, leaf or bag	1 cup/8 ounces/237 ml	50 mg
Tea, decaffeinated	1 cup/8 ounces/237 ml	0 mg
Cola, regular	1 can/12 ounces/355 ml	36–46 mg
Cola, diet	1 can/12 ounces/355 ml	39–50 mg
Chocolate milk	1 cup/8 ounces/237 ml	8 mg
Hot cocoa, 1 envelope	1 cup/8 ounces/237 ml	5 mg
Candy, milk chocolate	1 ounce/28 g (about 1/2 chocolate bar)	7 mg
Chocolate pudding	5.1 ounces/145 g	9 mg
Chocolate brownies	1.5 ounces/42 g	10 mg

Source: Adapted from Health Canada. "Caffeine in Food." (www.hc-sc.gc.ca/fn-an/securit/addit/caf/food-caf-aliments-eng.php)

almost trivial, though, once again, the study designs varied considerably, so it's hard to say for sure just how big an effect green tea could really have in the long run.

Green Tea and Cancer

Green tea has long been associated with a reduced risk of cancer. Unfortunately, cancer is probably the most difficult of the three most prominent Western diseases (cancer, type 2 diabetes, and heart disease) to study; it simply doesn't have the same surrogate markers to measure risk, as with high blood sugar for diabetes and high blood pressure for heart disease. As a result, much of the available research uses retrospective population studies, which means researchers look at the dietary habits of a group of people who developed cancer and then try to find links to these habits and the subjects' health. Although these studies are useful for suggesting a relationship between a behaviour (green tea consumption) and an outcome (cancer risk), they don't tell us if one actually causes the other.

Nonetheless, based on several meta-analyses, green tea may be associated with a reduced risk of prostate cancer, especially in Asian populations,[80] as well as ovarian and endometrial cancers,[81]

RECOMMENDED MAXIMUM CAFFEINE INTAKE

GROUP	RECOMMENDED MAXIMUM CAFFEINE INTAKE
Children 4–6 years	45 mg/day
Children 7–9 years	62.5 mg/day
Children 10–12 years	85 mg/day
Teens 13–17 years	No definitive recommendation because of insufficient data; recommended maximum intake of 2.5 mg/kg body weight
Women who are planning to become pregnant, pregnant women, and breastfeeding mothers	300 mg/day
Adults	400 mg/day

Source: Adapted from Health Canada. "Caffeine in Food." (www.hc-sc.gc.ca/fn-an/securit/addit/caf/food-caf-aliments-eng.php)

liver cancer,[82] and breast cancer recurrence and possibly incidence.[83] To date, however, no studies have demonstrated a cause and effect between green tea and cancer; these results could simply be because those who drink green tea also make other lifestyle choices that reduce their risk of the disease.

BREWING THE BEST CUP OF TEA

Green tea has different properties than black tea, and as such, it should be prepared in its own way. To brew green tea properly, it is generally recommended to use water that is below boiling; too hot and you will destroy much of the flavour, possibly by liberating more tannins from the tea, compounds that not only deliver a bitter taste but might also bind calcium and iron. Ideally, fresh green tea leaves should be kept in an airtight container to keep them from oxidizing (going rancid), and the brewing time is usually kept to about three minutes or less— much less than black tea. Green tea is generally taken without milk or sugar, and there is some evidence that adding milk or soy beverage can reduce some of green tea's benefits by reducing the availability of catechins.[84]

THE BOTTOM LINE

As one of the most-studied foods on earth, it is a bit disappointing to not have more confidence in the results we have to date on green tea. Even so, it is intriguing that a drink with no nutritional value per se seems to have a small but seemingly genuine effect on blood sugar levels, cancer risk, and possibly even cholesterol and weight. As with coffee, one must be mindful of the caffeine content of green tea, but if you enjoy it and can tolerate it well, then why not reap its benefits, even if they are relatively small?

OATS

Remember oats? Before the term *superfood* had ever been uttered, oats were one of the earliest health foods. With research on heart health benefits dating back to the 1960s, oats have long been associated with middle-aged guys with cholesterol problems. Although this image might have made oats seem like the breakfast of bores, oatmeal is thankfully enjoying a second run in the spotlight as healthy living takes centre stage. This time, however, oats must compete for our warm-breakfast attention with the likes of buckwheat, quinoa, and amaranth while straining under its at-times confusing gluten-free status. But does the competition with newer, ultra-cool grains mean oats have become the nutrition equivalent of the VHS tape? Not at all: Oats might not be the only whole grain option out there, but they remain one of the best—and are by far the best studied. In fact, the more we learn about oats, the more impressive they become.

OATS: THE STORY

Oats, or *Avena sativa*, are a member of the Poaceae family, meaning that, unlike quinoa, amaranth, and buckwheat, they are a true cereal grain. Popular as porridge, in mixed breakfast cereals, or as an ingredient in baked goods and snack foods, oats are actually most commonly used to feed livestock, not humans. In England, oats served for centuries as fine dining for horses, but their capacity to tolerate cooler, rainier climates meant they eventually became a popular crop and nutritional staple for the Scottish and Irish people. According to Samuel Johnson's 1755 *Dictionary of the English Language*, oats are defined as "a grain, which in England is generally given to horses, but in Scotland appears to support the people."[85] It's been said the Scots would then reply, "That's why England has such great horses, and Scotland has such fine men!"[86]

OATS: THE NUTRITION

Oats are one of the lowest-calorie grains: A cup of cooked oats (234 grams) provides 166 calories' worth of energy, about a hundred less than comparable volumes of cooked amaranth or quinoa. You'll also pick up 6 grams of protein and 4 grams of fibre from a cup of oatmeal (targets for dietary fibre range from 25 to 38 grams per day for an average adult). Lower in most B vitamins than quinoa or amaranth, oats are still one of the richest grain sources of vitamin B_1, which is important for turning carbohydrates into energy, providing 12% of your daily needs (quinoa provides 13%, while amaranth provides only 2%). Likewise, while oats are lower in magnesium than some other whole grains (providing 16% of your daily requirements versus 30% for a cup of cooked quinoa), they still provide a respectable 12% of your iron, 16% of your zinc, 18% of your selenium, and 9% of your daily copper needs.

OATS: THE SCIENCE

Oats are one of the best-researched foods of any kind. Let's take a look at just a sampling of the available research.

Oats and Cholesterol

The ability of oats to lower both total and the so-called bad (LDL) cholesterol is well established. The key nutrient appears to be beta-glucan, a type of fibre present in both oats and barley. Beta-glucan is from the family of fibres known as soluble fibre, which is believed to prevent the body from building new cholesterol while also binding cholesterol in the bowel, causing us to excrete it during our daily trip to the john. A recent meta-analysis found that a minimum of 3 grams of beta-glucan per day (about the amount you'll obtain from a bowl of cooked oatmeal) is needed to have a significant

SELECT NUTRIENTS IN WHOLE GRAINS AND PSEUDOCEREALS

ITEM	Oats	Quinoa	Amaranth
AMOUNT	1 cup, cooked (234 g)	1 cup, cooked (185 g)	1 cup, cooked (246 g)
Calories	166	222	251
Fat	4 g	4 g	4 g
Carbohydrate	32 g	39 g	46 g
Fibre	4 g	5 g	5 g
Protein	6 g	8 g	9 g
Vitamin B$_1$	12%	13%	2%
Vitamin B$_2$	2%	12%	3%
Vitamin B$_3$	3%	4%	3%
Vitamin B$_6$	1%	11%	14%
Folate	4%	19%	14%
Calcium	2%	3%	12%
Iron	12%	15%	29%
Magnesium	16%	30%	40%
Potassium	5%	9%	9%
Zinc	16%	13%	14%
Selenium	18%	7%	19%

Source: USDA National Nutrient Database

impact on cholesterol, triggering a roughly 5% drop in total cholesterol and about a 7% drop in LDL cholesterol.[87] In absolute values, a similar meta-analysis found that beta-glucan triggered an average drop in LDL cholesterol of about 0.66 mmol/L.[88]

To put those numbers into context, an individual at a low risk of experiencing a cardiovascular event (technically defined as someone who has less than a 10% chance of experiencing a heart attack, stroke, or angina in the next 10 years, according to what is known as the

Framingham Risk Score) would be prescribed cholesterol-lowering medication if LDL cholesterol exceeds 5.0 mmol/L. Those at moderate risk (10% to 20% risk of experiencing a cardiovascular event in the next decade) are generally recommended medication when LDL exceeds 3.5, and high-risk individuals (with more than a 20% risk of a cardiac event in the next 10 years; that group automatically includes all people with type 2 diabetes) are recommended statin (cholesterol-lowering) drugs if their LDL exceeds 2.0 mmol/L. So, if the simple habit of eating oatmeal daily could bring a high-risk person's LDL cholesterol down from 2.6 to 2.0 mmol/L, that could be a substantial enough change to keep some people off of medication. The effect might not be the same in all individuals (the healthier your diet is to start, the less of an effect you'll usually see), but it emphasizes the fact that, sometimes, small changes to our habits can have a big effect on our health.

Oats and Blood Pressure

In addition to their cholesterol-lowering effect, oats may help with blood pressure control, possibly through either their fibre or magnesium content or both. In one particularly well-designed study, published by researchers at the University of Aberdeen in 2010, 206 healthy adults of various weights were asked to substitute three servings of refined grain products (such as white bread, pasta, or rice) with either three servings per day of whole wheat products or one serving of whole wheat and two servings of oats per day. The control group were told to continue with their usual diets. At the end of 12 weeks, the subjects in both the whole wheat and the whole-wheat-plus-oats groups saw their systolic blood pressure (that's the top number) drop by between 5 and 6 points, a significant change versus those consuming the refined grains.[89] Amazingly, that effect on systolic blood pressure is not far off what is seen in those who cut their salt (sodium) intake from high to low: In the classic research on the Dietary Approaches to Stop Hypertension (DASH) diet (an eating plan that is rich in blood-pressure-lowering nutrients, such as calcium, magnesium, and potassium as well as fibre-rich foods), slashing sodium intake resulted in an average drop in systolic blood pressure of about 11 points in those with high blood pressure (hypertension) and by 7 points in those whose blood pressure was normal.[90] In other words, a person with normal blood pressure could see a similar drop in blood pressure by cutting sodium intake drastically or by substituting three servings of refined grains for whole grains and oats instead.

Oats and Blood Sugar

Although some studies on adults without diabetes suggest that oats may improve blood sugar control, the results have been inconsistent.[91] In one interesting study on people with type 2 diabetes admitted to hospital because of very poor blood sugar control, daily consumption of oats substantially improved glycemic (blood sugar) control, as well as reliance on insulin as medication, within just a few days, an effect that was even more pronounced than if they had been put on a traditional diabetes diet.[92]

WHAT'S BETTER: STEEL-CUT OR INSTANT OATS?

With a sweeter taste than many grains, oats have made a popular breakfast cereal for centuries. Although the majority of oats contain both the nutrient-dense bran and germ, the oats themselves may be flattened (rolled) and steamed to help speed cooking. This process results in instant or quick-cooking rolled oats, which may be prepared in as little as one minute with boiling water. On the other hand, whole oats kernels, also known as groats, that have been sliced once or twice to allow water to access the grain for cooking are often called steel-cut or Irish oats. These oats require significantly longer cooking times (about 20 to 30 minutes) but have a nuttier, slightly crunchy taste that many people enjoy. The difference between the two, nutritionally speaking, isn't hugely significant, but there may be a slight effect on glycemic, or blood sugar, response: Although instant oats (such as Quaker one-minute oats) have a glycemic index (GI) of about 66 (the glycemic index refers to the capacity of different foods to raise blood sugar, usually compared with pure glucose sugar), putting them in the moderate glycemic range (a food with a GI of 56 to 69, compared with pure glucose's GI of 100, is considered moderate GI), slower-cooking oats have a GI in the low to mid-50s, putting them in the range of low-GI foods. The lesser blood sugar effect could not only be useful for people with diabetes who need to control their blood sugar but could also help healthy individuals feel full longer, and healthy blood sugar control might reduce their risk of chronic disease, especially type 2 diabetes, in the long run.[93]

Oats and Cancer

A small but intriguing body of evidence suggests that oats could have an anticancer effect. So far, most of the data is in cell lines or animal studies, but a handful of studies conducted in Asia suggest beta-glucan could extend survival rates and quality of life in those who have been diagnosed with cancer.[94] Cell line studies also suggest that compounds unique to oats, known as avenanthramides (try saying *that* three times fast), may protect against the proliferation of colon cancer cells.[95] Unfortunately, since there is little research in this area, we don't yet have an idea of an optimal dose of oats or beta-glucan that could exert a benefit for prevention or treatment of cancer, but it at least suggests that this is an area to watch.

Oats and Dry Skin and Eczema

Although much of the research on food relates to its benefits for our insides, oats are a relatively uncommon food that has also been studied for its effect on our outsides—namely, our skin. Oats used in a liquid suspension, known as colloidal oatmeal, have a long history of use as a treatment for dry skin and eczema, also known as atopic dermatitis. The oatmeal not only acts as a natural moisturizer but also reduces inflammation and improves the skin's natural barriers, which is important for minimizing the redness, itching, and cracking associated with eczema. A 2012 review conducted by researchers at the University of Louisville suggested that colloidal oatmeal can help reduce itchiness, dryness, and the amount of area affected for those with mild to moderate eczema for individuals of all ages, including infants and children.[96]

Oats and Asthma

The timing of early food introduction for infants is thought to influence allergy, asthma, and eczema risk later in life. Although many public health agencies recommend exclusive breastfeeding for six months, there is some data to suggest that introducing certain foods before six months might actually be protective against allergies and associated conditions. In recent years, a group of Finnish researchers have examined this relationship in several studies and have found that introducing oats between 5 and 5.5 months of age may be associated with a lower incidence of asthma later in childhood.[97, 98]

ARE OATS GLUTEN FREE?

Although oats were once thought to contain gluten, it is now understood that they do not; instead, it is cross-contamination with wheat, barley, or other gluten-containing grains that seems to trigger symptoms in those with celiac disease or the more recently defined non-celiac gluten sensitivity. Since the threshold for a food to be considered gluten free is very small (just 20 parts per million, or ppm), even the presence of other gluten-containing grains in the same facility as oats could often result in enough contamination with gluten to trigger symptoms in affected individuals. Fortunately, a handful of oat producers have taken steps to bring gluten-free oats to market, piggybacking on the Canadian Celiac Association's 2007 Position Statement on Oats, which states that "consumption of pure, uncontaminated oats is safe in the amount of 50 to 70 grams per day (1/2 to 3/4 cup dry rolled oats) by adults and 20 to 25 grams per day (1/4 cup of dry rolled oats) by children with celiac disease."[99]

THE BOTTOM LINE

Oatmeal might be the breakfast your grandma (or great-grandma) ate, but that doesn't mean it's passé. With potential health benefits ranging from cholesterol control to asthma prevention, oats and oatmeal have plenty to offer. Although perhaps not providing the same broad spectrum of nutrients as the likes of quinoa or amaranth, oats differ from the pseudocereals in their beta-glucan content, giving them a unique nutrition profile. So, whether it's a warm bowl of porridge on a cold winter morning or a cup of cold overnight oats in the heat of the summer, there is good reason to include one of nature's best cereal grains in your diet, both now and presumably for many years to come.

KALE

"In this day and age when the average person may feel too busy to exercise, relax or take the time to eat well, when families are struggling to create fast yet healthy meals within a budget, and everyone is looking for a way to boost their immunity, kale just seems too good to be true." So begins the preface of Sharon Hanna's *The Book of Kale*.[100] Those are some strong words, but how true are they?

KALE: THE STORY

Kale (*Brassica oleracea*, variety *acephala*) is a dark-green, leafy vegetable that grows easily in many different climates. A part of the same *Brassica* family that includes cabbage, broccoli, and cauliflower, kale has a long history of use in many cultures and was reportedly part of the burial process in Ancient Egypt. Fossil records also suggest that kale-like plants may have existed in prehistoric times, dating as far back as the time of dinosaurs.

A hardy vegetable, kale can tolerate cool spring weather, the heat of summer, and even frost, after which it actually becomes sweeter tasting. It grows well in many conditions, and while it ideally needs a fair amount of sun, kale requires less water than many other garden plants. All of these circumstances, plus kale's impressive nutrient offerings, make it a popular choice for both gardeners and the health-minded alike.

KALE: THE NUTRITION

When you hear the claim that kale might well be the mother of all superfoods, it makes sense to be a bit skeptical. After all, there are many green and orange veggies, not to mention berries, nuts, seeds, and pulses, as well as oily fish, that could all vie for the title.

Calorie-wise, kale provides a mere 33 calories per cup, uncooked, which, although low, is not as low as spinach (7 calories per cup). Although its protein (2 grams), carbohydrate (7 grams), and even fibre content (1 gram) aren't worthy of bragging rights, kale's vitamin and mineral content are, quite frankly, astonishing: That same 1-cup serving provides over 200% of your daily vitamin A requirements, 134% of vitamin C, and a stunning 700% of vitamin K. Did you read that right? Yes, a cup of raw kale has more vitamin C than an orange and more vitamin A than a carrot. And there's really nothing that compares on the vitamin K front, except for a handful of other dark green vegetables. Kale is also a source (providing at least 5%) of numerous B vitamins, particularly vitamin B_6, and of iron and magnesium, and it provides about 300 mg of potassium per serving.

But what if you eat your kale cooked? Does that destroy all the good nutrition? As with many vegetables, steaming or sautéing kale changes its profile somewhat, but the numbers are still worthy of our attention: Although the vitamin C content of a cup of boiled kale declines to 89% of your daily requirement, its vitamin K content doubles (to about 1,400%), as does its vitamin A, which also becomes more bioavailable, which means it is better able to be used by the body. The reason for this spike in nutrient content? It's simply a matter of volume: When you cook kale—or any other leafy green—it shrinks down by a significant amount, which means you'll pack an awful lot more kale into a 1-cup serving.

Kale has also garnered some attention for its calcium content, which amounts to just under 100 mg, or about 10% of an adult's daily requirements, per cup, raw or cooked. Although that isn't necessarily a mind-blowing number, kale is low in oxalates, compounds that are known to bind various nutrients, including calcium, causing them to be excreted in our urine. Although other higher-oxalate vegetables, such as spinach, are known to have poor calcium absorbability,[101] research conducted by Dr. Robert Heaney, an expert in calcium metabolism, and colleagues has demonstrated that, gram for gram, the calcium from kale is absorbed at least as well as the calcium from milk.[102] The same is likely also true for other lower-oxalate vegetables, including broccoli, turnip, and mustard greens.

Kale's uber–vitamin K status means it is probably not a great choice for people on blood thinners, as it will counteract some of the effect of the medication. Kale has also recently garnered some negative press because it, along with collard greens, has earned a spot on the Environmental Working Group's Dirty Dozen Plus list of foods most likely to be contaminated with pesticides, especially compounds known as organophosphates that, while being withdrawn from use, still exist in soil.[103] As a result, the EWG recommends that kale and other leafy greens be purchased as organic whenever possible.

Kale can be enjoyed raw or cooked, in mixed dishes, or as a side dish on its own. One of the most popular options is the kale chip, which, despite what your kids or dad might believe, are not only tasty but also totally addictive. Kale or baby (young) kale also works well as a salad ingredient, in stir-fries and omelettes, and sautéed with garlic, onions, and a bit of olive oil. If you are prepping a meal rich in vitamin K, be it from kale, chard, collard greens, asparagus, or other green vegetables, you might consider adding a bit of fat to the meal, be it through olive oil, avocado, nuts, seeds, or even a touch of butter: Research has demonstrated that, while only a small fraction of the vitamin K we eat makes it into our bodies, that quantity increases significantly when we eat it with some fat.[104]

KALE: THE SCIENCE

Perhaps the most significant nutrient found in kale is vitamin K. Vitamin K is a particularly intriguing nutrient that has flown under the radar, so let's take a closer look.

As with many vitamins, including vitamin A and vitamin E, vitamin K isn't just a single compound; instead, it exists in numerous forms both in food and in our bodies. As mentioned in the discussion on cheese, there are two main types of vitamin K: phylloquinone (FIE-low-kwin-own), or vitamin K_1, which occurs in plant foods, especially kale, collard greens, parsley, and Swiss chard, and menaquinones (of which there are several), or vitamin K_2, which exist in cheese, animal foods, and the Japanese fermented soy food natto. For the purposes of this discussion, we'll focus on vitamin K_1, which is found in such large amounts in kale.

Vitamin K and Blood Clotting

Among its many actions in the human body, the best-known and best-studied role for vitamin K is in healthy blood clotting; in fact, the German term *Koagulation* was the genesis for the vitamin's moniker. Specifically, vitamin K's job is to help the clotting factors, of which there are several (usually expressed in Roman numerals, such as clotting factor VI), to "stick" to the cells that surround an area that has been wounded. Without vitamin K, your body couldn't stop a paper cut from turning into a full-blown hemorrhage, and we would bleed out from even minor injuries. It's also this objective—to stop clotting—that forms the foundation of our use of anticoagulant medications, including Coumadin (also known by its generic name, warfarin). Although healthy clotting activity is a good thing, some individuals are at risk of too much clotting, which can be a trigger for a stroke or other cardiac event. In that case, they may be prescribed the drug Coumadin to keep their blood flowing freely and are often advised to cut back on vitamin K–rich foods to allow the medication to work effectively.

Vitamin K and Bone Health

Aside from vitamin K's role in clotting, it is also fairly well known for being an important factor in bone health. Although one might imagine bones as static objects, like stones, in reality, they are very dynamic. At any given moment, our bones are either building up or breaking down, and in fact, both processes occur at once; it's just a question of which side of the equation is winning (this is similar to what happens in our muscles). A key player in the bone break-down process—which is necessary so that your body can liberate calcium for other important functions—is a cell known as an osteo-clast. Osteoclasts are bone demineralizers; they take calcium from the bone, and while that's not a bad thing in small amounts, it can become a problem if their work outpaces the efforts of their coun-terparts, osteoblasts, whose job it is to build bones back up. Both osteoclasts and osteoblasts, it turns out, are affected by vitamin K status, as is a protein produced by osteoblasts, known as osteocalcin. When you eat a vitamin K–rich meal (such as kale), the phylloqui-none gets calcitonin ready for action through a process known as car-boxylation. Once osteocalcin has been carboxylated, it then signals the osteoblasts that it's time to go to work, and your body responds by going into bone-building mode.[105] Without vitamin K, then, our osteocalcin would be left undercarboxylated (undercarboxylated osteocalcin is actually an increasingly well-accepted measure for inadequate vitamin K status), and our osteoblasts wouldn't do their job. The results, over time, could be weaker bones and, eventually, an increased risk of osteoporosis.

· ·

TOP SUPERFOOD SOURCES OF VITAMIN K

FOOD	PORTION	VITAMIN K	VITAMIN K (% DAILY VALUE)
Kale	1 cup, raw (67 g)	547 mcg	684%
Collard greens	1 cup, raw (36 g)	184 mcg	230%
Spinach	1 cup, raw (30 g)	145 mcg	181%
Broccoli	1 cup, raw (91 g)	93 mcg	116%
Kiwi	2 large fruit, without skin (182 g)	74 mcg	92%
Avocados	1 cup, cubed (150 g)	32 mcg	39%
Blueberries, cultivated	1 cup (148 g)	29 mcg	36%
Pomegranate	1 cup arils (176 g)	28 mcg	36%
Pumpkin seeds	1 ounce (28 g)	13 mcg	17%

Source: USDA National Nutrient Database

Vitamin K, Blood Sugar, and Metabolic Syndrome

Beyond its effect on bones and blood, an interesting new line of evidence suggests that vitamin K could play a role in our ability to regulate blood sugar and possibly protect us against metabolic syndrome, the cluster of symptoms associated with an increased risk of type 2 diabetes and heart disease.[106] Studies on rats fed a diet low in vitamin K_1 (phylloquinone) found their blood sugar began to drift higher, and they became less responsive to the hormone insulin, whose job it is to control blood sugar. In humans, the results of the Framingham Offspring Study (the Framingham Heart Study, which followed a group of people from Framingham, Massachusetts, for decades, is perhaps the most significant study of cardiovascular risk factors ever conducted; the Offspring Study is following their children) found that, among 2,719 men and women, higher intakes of vitamin K_1 were associated with better insulin sensitivity and improved blood sugar levels.[107] Although researchers don't yet know why or how this is the case—and it's possible that vitamin K could just be a marker of a healthier diet or lifestyle overall[108] (though the researchers do try to control for those possibilities), we now know that both phylloquinone (vitamin K_1) and one of the forms of vitamin K_2, known as MK_4, are found in the pancreas, the organ responsible for producing insulin. It has also been found that osteocalcin, the bone-building protein activated by phylloquinone, could make our bodies more sensitive to insulin and help the pancreas do its work.

Finally, there is a small but intriguing body of evidence suggesting that vitamin K reduces inflammation in the body by reducing levels of particular cytokines, or mini-hormones, that trigger inflammation.[109] High levels of inflammation in the body, which can be made worse by weight gain and poor diet, are associated with poor insulin sensitivity and increased risk of type 2 diabetes, so it's possible that vitamin K can play a role in preventing not only diabetes but also many other conditions that are inflammation mediated, including heart disease.

PREPARING KALE CHIPS

To prepare kale chips, simply wash and dry a bushel of fresh kale and then chop it into small segments—about 1 to 2 inches in length and width—discarding any hard, bony stems. Line a pair of cookie trays with parchment or wax paper, and spread the kale pieces out so that none of the kale overlaps. Brush olive oil lightly over the kale, then sprinkle with sea or kosher salt. Add extra flavour via soy sauce or tamari if you wish. Bake at 325°F for about 10 to 15 minutes, bearing in mind that the objective is not to burn the leaves but to dry them out.[110]

THE BOTTOM LINE

Easy to grow, hardy, and nutrient dense, kale is a great choice for gardeners both young and old. Getting kids involved helps foster a sense of connection to food and an understanding of where it comes from, and it may also make them more likely to eat it. As for its super-food status? Based on vitamin K alone, not to mention the rest of its chart-topping vitamin A, C, and calcium profile, it's hard to argue that kale doesn't deserve a spot at, or near, the top of any superfood list.

STRAWBERRIES

Come on, who doesn't love strawberries? Cute, red, and sweet, we might intuitively know that strawberries are good for us, but it's only in recent years that we've begun to understand just how significant their contribution to our health could be.

STRAWBERRIES: THE STORY

Technically speaking, strawberries (*Fragaria* × *ananassa*), a member of the Rosaceae, or rose, family, are not actually berries. In the realm of plant biology, berries are the ripened fleshy parts of the ovary of a female plant, which is where you would find the seeds. By that defi-nition, tomatoes, bananas, avocados, and even watermelons are all berries. In more common language, however, we tend to think of any small, delicate fruit as a berry, so strawberries are often placed in the same category as "real" berries, such as blueberries, cranberries, and currants (note that raspberries and blackberries are also not botan-ical berries).

Fossil evidence suggests that strawberries have existed in Europe since prehistoric times, and the fruit and boiled leaves have been used for medicinal purposes for centuries. Strawberries were first cultivated in England in the 1600s and eventually in North America by the 19th century, although early settlers, including the explorer Jacques Cartier, found the wild berries along the St. Lawrence River in Canada long before then. Although strawberries are now grown all over North America, in Canada they are usually available fresh in June and July, though everbearing cultivars will produce berries twice per year, with the second wave available through August and early September. In the United States, nearly 90% of strawberries are grown and harvested in the state of California, and we northerners certainly take advantage: Canadians eat more strawberries per year than all other berries combined.[111]

STRAWBERRIES: THE NUTRITION

A cup of sliced (halved) strawberries (152 grams) provides a mere 49 calories—less than both blueberries and blackberries. Strawberries' fibre content, however, is also the lowest of the three, at 3 grams per serving (blueberries offer up 4 grams and blackberries 8, by comparison). Perhaps one of the least-appreciated nutrition facts about strawberries is their vitamin C content: A cup of fresh berries provides 149% of your vitamin C for the day—that's more than you'll get from a cup of orange juice. Vitamin C aside, however, strawberries are also a source (providing more than 5% of your daily requirements) of folate, magnesium, and potassium, but they score above the 10% level for only one nutrient, the ever-present manganese. In other words, when it comes to their basic nutrient composition, strawberries score top marks for weight management (because of their low calorie content) and vitamin C more than anything else. Although strawberries do contain sugar, their impact on blood sugar is very limited: With a glycemic index (GI) of 40, strawberries rank as a low-glycemic food.[112]

STRAWBERRIES: THE SCIENCE

Strawberries are a rare fruit with a well-established body of research. Several well-controlled human studies have been conducted on strawberries, many with promising results.

Strawberries and Heart Health

In a 2010 study published by a group of Oklahoma-based researchers, the same group that has also published studies on the impact of blueberries on heart health, 27 overweight and obese men and women with metabolic syndrome found that consuming a daily strawberry drink, equivalent to 3 cups of strawberries per day, for eight weeks, helped lower their total cholesterol from 5.8 to 5.2 mmol/L and their LDL cholesterol from 3.5 to 3.1 mmol/L. Since an LDL of 3.5 mmol/L is the threshold for placing an individual at moderate risk of heart attack, stroke, or angina on cholesterol-lowering drugs, the results suggest that strawberries could play a significant role in heart health.[113]

In another study, the same Toronto-based group studying the effect of the portfolio diet of cholesterol-lowering foods gave subjects who had already been following the diet, which is based on soluble fibre, soy, plant sterols, and nuts, an additional pound (454 grams) of strawberries and compared the effects with a group of people taking an equal number of calories from oat bran bread (remember, oat bran is known for cholesterol-lowering effects). After a month, the groups switched. Sure enough, the strawberries proved equally effective to oat bran in controlling LDL cholesterol, but the LDL of the strawberry eaters showed less oxidative damage (thought to be a trigger for the development of plaques) than those taking the oat bran bread.[114] Now, although this study used a dose of strawberries that isn't sustainable for most, it still piques the interest to see how well strawberries fared against other titans of cholesterol control, such as oat bran.

Beyond total and LDL cholesterol, strawberries also might be able to mitigate some of the short-term damage to our LDL cholesterol that occurs after we indulge in a greasy meal.[115] Strawberries also seem to shift our LDL ("bad") cholesterol toward large, fluffy LDL cholesterol, which is considered less harmful to the heart, while also reducing the number of small particles of HDL, a fraction of the so-called good cholesterol that may not be so good for us.[116] The bottom line? Strawberries might exert their heart health effect on cholesterol not only in the big picture but also in less-obvious ways that might be just as important.

Strawberries and Cancer

Strawberries contain a compound known as fisetin, which is thought to have anticancer properties. Cell studies have demonstrated that fisetin, which comes from a family of plant-based compounds known as flavonols, inhibits two chemical pathways, one known as PI3K/Akt and the other known as mTOR.[117] Although activation of these pathways is important for a number of basic cellular functions—the mTOR pathway, for example, helps initiate the process of building new muscle tissue after a workout—these pathways may be overly active in some types of tumours. For that reason, compounds that can suppress both PI3K/Akt and mTOR have shown promise as potential therapies for cancer treatment.

There is enough interest in the anticancer potential of strawberries that a Chinese-American research team is conducting drug-like trials of the effect of freeze-dried strawberry powder on precancerous lesions in the throat (esophagus). In the most recent study, published in 2012, a group of 75 patients with precancerous throat lesions were given either 30 grams or 60 grams of strawberry powder each day. After six months, the lesions of those receiving the lower dose were unchanged, but 80% of the subjects in the higher-dose group saw the degree of severity of their lesions decline.[118]

HOW DO YOU TAKE YOUR STRAWBERRIES?

Strawberries should be washed gently before serving, but be careful not to soak them, as they will absorb water and lose flavour. Frozen strawberries retain much but not all of their vitamin C content, and while their tender skin is easily damaged with freezing, they still work well in mixed dishes, such as smoothies, and can be enjoyed frozen as a snack.

Unfortunately, concern has been raised over the pesticide content of strawberries, along with other soft-skinned fruits and vegetables. The U.S.-based Environmental Working Agency has consistently listed strawberries among their "dirty dozen" fruits and vegetables most likely to be contaminated with pesticides, even after washing.[119] A recent study, published in the journal *Environmental Health*, found that strawberries were among the foods most likely to contribute to pesticides in the diets of preschool and school-aged children in California.[120]

THE BOTTOM LINE

For all the hype afforded to blueberries, it is the strawberry that is arguably backed by a better body of research. With some good evidence that strawberries can help lower cholesterol and other factors associated with heart disease, we can all be thankful that the little red berry that makes our summers more enjoyable might have just as much, if not more, to offer our health as superfoods from jungles far away.

SPINACH

Popeye ate spinach to make him strong. So, it must be good, right? No doubt, spinach, one of the most well-known and commonly used dark green vegetables, has a place in the pantheon of superveggies. But how does it stack up against the likes of kale? And what of the notion that spinach can make you strong (or, as my grandfather liked to say, "put hair on your chest")? Let's take a closer look.

SPINACH: THE STORY

Spinach (*Spinacia oleracea*) is a member of the goosefoot, or Chenopodiaceae, family. Although spinach grows well in cooler weather, much like broccoli, spinach's origins have been traced back to the warmer climate of Persia (now Iran). By the 1300s, spinach was being cultivated in Europe and Britain, and it made its way to North America by the early 1800s. In the 1930s, a sailor named Popeye brought fame to this dark green vegetable by claiming that eating spinach made him strong. Although exactly what part of spinach is thought to have conferred Popeye his legendary strength is a matter of debate (some say it was the iron, while a revisionist version of events says it was actually its vitamin A content), but there's little doubt that Popeye was doing himself some good by eating it.

SPINACH: THE NUTRITION

In terms of calorie content, there are few foods as low as spinach: A cup (30 grams) of uncooked spinach provides a puny 7 calories, which means you probably burn more calories making a spinach salad than eating it. Since its calorie content is so low, it is also low in all the macronutrients (protein, carbohydrate, and fat) and contains a slim 1 gram of fibre.

In terms of vitamin and mineral content, raw spinach provides about half a day's vitamin A (as beta-carotene—56%) and nearly two days' worth of vitamin K (181%), which, although fantastic in its own right, does fall behind kale and collard greens. A cup of raw spinach also provides 14% of your daily vitamin C, 6% of your magnesium, 5% of your iron and potassium, and 15% of your folate needs.

On the other hand, once you cook spinach, the volume shrinks down so much that you suddenly find yourself packing in a lot more nutrients in a smaller space. A 1/2 cup of cooked (boiled, specifically) frozen spinach, for example, provides 32 calories, 4 grams of fibre, 229% of your daily vitamin A, and 642% of your daily vitamin K requirements. It is a source (meaning it provides more than 5% of your daily needs) of calcium, iron, and vitamin B_2; a good source (meaning it provides more than 15% of your daily needs) of vitamin E and magnesium; and an excellent source (meaning it provides more than 25% of your daily needs) of folate. Much of the reason for the more impressive numbers relates to the amount of spinach you're actually consuming: 1 cup of raw spinach is equal to about 30 grams, but 1/2 cup of cooked spinach is about 95 grams.

Beyond vitamins and minerals, spinach is also a rich food source of lutein, a type of carotenoid thought to be important for eye health. In a 1998 study examining the lutein content of various fruits and vegetables, spinach ranked as the seventh-richest source of lutein, behind egg yolk, corn, kiwi, red seedless grapes, zucchini, and pumpkin.[121] As with many foods, there is evidence that eating spinach with a source of fat can improve absorption of certain nutrients, lutein being one. Interestingly, a 2012 study conducted by French researchers found that spinach with butter or palm oil—both rich in saturated fats that have long been deemed unhealthy for the heart—raised circulating levels of lutein in rats better than olive oil or fish oil.[122]

Unlike kale, spinach contains oxalates, a type of naturally occurring salt that can bind certain nutrients and cause them to be excreted in our urine. This is particularly an issue for calcium, which is poorly absorbed from spinach.[123] Bagged spinach has also been associated with salmonella outbreaks, but interestingly, a recent study found that adding canola oil and vinegar to raw spinach (as you would in a salad) destroys much of the salmonella.[124] Nonetheless, you're still well advised to give all your veggies a good rinse before eating, even if they do say they are prewashed.

SPINACH: THE SCIENCE

Spinach is one of the richest food sources of nitrates, which, as we learned with beets, might not be the health hazard we once thought. Nitrates, if you recall, are converted to nitrite by the healthy bacteria in our mouths and are then made into nitric oxide, which seems to have far-reaching effects throughout our bodies, helping to decrease our blood pressure and increase our ability to tolerate strenuous exercise.[125, 126] A recent randomized controlled trial by Australian researchers also found that eating nitrate-rich spinach triggered an immediate improvement in what is known as flow-mediated dilation, or blood flow, through our arteries.[127]

SPINACH FOR GREEN SMOOTHIES

If you haven't tried it yet, you can easily add fresh or frozen spinach to your next smoothie—it is amazing how it disappears into the taste of the banana or apple. Try adding a handful of fresh spinach (taking the stems off is great, if you have the time), baby spinach (young spinach, which has a milder taste), or chunks of frozen spinach the next time you're making a breakfast smoothie or post-workout shake—you'll be surprised by the new way you can enjoy these age-old greens.

THE BOTTOM LINE

Spinach is a classic superfood, and it's not going away anytime fast. A great complement to kale, broccoli, chard, and other green veggies, spinach brings its own unique qualities to both your diet and your kitchen and is perhaps the most versatile of all the leafy greens when it comes to meal prep and palatability.

SWEET POTATOES

Once upon a time, we ate potatoes, and lots of them. Then, somewhere along the line, potatoes got a bad name. Being the opportunists they are, sweet potatoes seized the day and surprised many along the way when it was claimed they have a lower impact on blood sugar than regular potatoes, along with a more impressive nutrition profile.

(And, then, of course, came the sweet potato fries . . .)

SWEET POTATOES: THE STORY

Sweet potatoes (*Ipomoea batatas*) have long served as a staple food for indigenous populations in Central and South America, Africa, and the Caribbean, as well as for Hawaiians, Papua New Guineans, and the Maori in New Zealand. Rich in beta-carotene, a precursor of vitamin A, sweet potatoes continue to be used the world over to help prevent deficiency in at-risk populations.

Sweet potatoes exist in a variety of colours, ranging from light yellow to deep orange to purple. Purple sweet potatoes and their leaves have received some attention for their anthocyanin content, the pigment responsible for the deep hue of blueberries and that has been associated with reduced disease risk and improved antioxidant status.[128] In Canada, the growing praise for the sweet potato has triggered a change in our eating habits: Our national intake of this starchy vegetable doubled between 2006 and 2010, but our intake of white potatoes still outnumbers them by 20 to 1.[129]

SWEET POTATOES: THE NUTRITION

A cup (200 grams) of sweet potato, baked with the skin on, clocks in at 180 calories, putting it somewhere in the middle compared with other starchy vegetables and grains. That same 1-cup serving provides 4 grams of protein and an impressive 7 grams of fibre. It does contain 13 grams of sugar, but as mentioned, it's been said that those sugars do not tend to translate into a rapid spike in blood glucose, as long as you don't overdo it.

Although sweet potatoes' macronutrient breakdown is impressive, their vitamin and mineral content is even better. A 1-cup serving provides a whopping 769% of your daily vitamin A—a number equalled only by few other foods—along with two-thirds of your vitamin C and 8% of your calcium and iron requirements. Sweet potatoes are a source of most B vitamins, providing more than 10% of your daily needs for vitamins B_1, B_2, and B_3 and nearly 30% of your needs for vitamin B_6. Their mineral content is also impressive: In addition to the iron and calcium, you'll obtain 14% of your magnesium (not as high as many whole grains, but still good) and a dazzling 27%—or 950 mg—of the potassium your body needs to help it function properly and control your blood pressure. There is no single food commonly consumed by North Americans that is as rich in potassium as sweet potatoes, and since it is estimated that only 4% of Americans meet their potassium needs every day (Canadians may fare a little better, but not much), it's clear that sweet potatoes can go a long way to helping you meet your needs for not only potassium but a wide variety of other nutrients, as well.

Since sweet potatoes do come in so many forms and colours, there could be variability in their nutritional status. To that point, as with numerous carotenoid-containing foods, there is evidence that taking sweet potatoes with some fat (olive oil, for example) increases the absorption of vitamin A.[130]

TOP SUPERFOOD SOURCES OF VITAMIN A

FOOD	PORTION	VITAMIN A	VITAMIN A (% DAILY VALUE)
Sweet potato	1 cup, baked in skin (200 g)	38,433 IU	769%
Kale	1 cup, raw (67 g)	10,302 IU	206%
Goji berries	30 g	~	140%
Spinach	1 cup, raw (30 g)	2,813 IU	56%
Collard greens	1 cup, raw (36 g)	2,400 IU	48%
Broccoli	1 cup, raw (91 g)	567 IU	11%

Source: USDA National Nutrient Database (all except goji berries, retrieved from navitasnaturals.com/product/449/Goji-Berries.html; ~ = data not available)

SWEET POTATOES: THE SCIENCE
Sweet Potatoes and Blood Sugar
The majority of research on sweet potatoes relates to their potential to improve blood sugar control in people with type 2 diabetes. To date, three randomized controlled trials, all from the same lab, have been conducted on the effects of an extract from white-skinned sweet

potatoes (4 grams/day) versus a placebo on blood sugar control in people with type 2 diabetes. At the end of the studies, which ranged from six weeks to five months, the subjects' average blood sugar control improved modestly, via a measure known as glycosylated hemoglobin, or HbA1c, which measures blood sugar control over a three-month period.[131, 132, 133] Unfortunately, although the data from these three trials looked promising, a review conducted by the *Cochrane Database of Systematic Reviews* in 2012 questioned the methodology of the studies, noting that overall, the risk of bias was "unclear or high."[134] What's more, despite all the hype around sweet potatoes' limited effect on blood sugar, repeated studies of its glycemic index (capacity to raise blood sugar versus plain glucose sugar) have actually found it to be highly variable, ranging from as low as 44 (anything under 55 is considered low) in some studies to a whopping 94 in one test of sweet potatoes that had been peeled and baked (as a reference, pure glucose sugar has a GI of 100).[135] Differences in type of sweet potato used, in the preparation method, or in quality of study design could explain some of these inconsistencies, but the bottom line is that the gap between sweet and white potatoes might not be as big as many have believed.

Sweet Potatoes and Blood Pressure

Although the connection between sweet potatoes and blood sugar may be more hype than substance, perhaps sweet potatoes' biggest bragging right is their potassium content. Potassium has long been associated with protection from high blood pressure, or hypertension, but early studies on potassium pills fizzled out. Then, in 1997, came a watershed moment, when the first paper on the Dietary Approaches to Stop Hypertension (DASH) diet was published in the *New England Journal of Medicine*.[136] In this large-scale study, conducted between 1994 and 1996, 502 generally healthy adults with high blood pressure, but not on medication, were first fed a diet low in fruits and vegetables with a fat content that mimicked the average American diet (this is called the run-in period, designed to make sure everyone is on equal footing at the start of the study). This lower-quality run-in diet (which, incidentally, triggered constipation in a number of the subjects) was designed to be low enough in key minerals associated with blood pressure control, particularly potassium, magnesium, and calcium, that the subjects fell into the bottom quarter of the average American intake.

From there, the unlucky subjects randomly assigned to the control group continued with the same diet, while one intervention group was given a diet rich in fruits and vegetables, designed to bring their potassium and magnesium intakes up to the level of the top quarter of Americans. A third group was given a diet rich in fruits, vegetables, and low-fat dairy products, which also brought their calcium up to the level of the top 25% of the population.

After eight weeks on the diet, which was prepared for the subjects to keep as much control over their eating as possible (they ate lunch and dinner at various study sites, then took home coolers with food for the rest of the day, as well as the next day's breakfast—this is an amazing level of control that has rarely been duplicated), the fruit/vegetable/dairy group (also known as the combination group) saw their blood pressure decrease by an average of 5.5/3.0 mm Hg more than those on the control diet. Those on the fruits and vegetables–only diet saw a drop in systolic blood pressure (top number) of 2.8 mm Hg and in diastolic blood pressure of 1.1 mm Hg (the bottom number).

Although those results, and the high quality of the study, certainly support the theory that potassium-, magnesium-, and calcium-rich foods can lower blood pressure, the results might look a little, well, modest. It bears mentioning, then, that the results include both those with normal blood pressure and those with hypertension. Since we wouldn't expect a huge change in the normal blood pressure group, what would happen if we looked only at those with high blood pressure? Now the data becomes all the more impressive: Their average blood pressure dropped by 11.4/5.5 mm Hg in the combination diet and by 7.2/2.8 mm Hg in the fruit and vegetable diet. Since the difference between healthy blood pressure (120/80) and hypertension (140/90) is relatively small, this suggests that, even without changing other blood pressure–affecting factors such as body weight, exercise, sodium, or alcohol intake, the simple act of eating more fruits, vegetables, and calcium-rich foods could potentially keep an awful lot of people off of blood pressure medication. In fact, the effects of the DASH diet are about as good as you'd get from putting someone on the first line of blood pressure medication. Pass the sweet potatoes, please.

Sweet Potatoes and Inflammation

In addition to their potential effects on blood sugar and blood pressure, sweet potatoes also possess anti-inflammatory properties, which could play a role in an array of diseases and medical conditions, ranging from heart disease to cancer to cognitive decline, although much more research is needed in this area. A recent review published in the journal *Toxicology and Industrial Health* suggested that sweet potatoes show some potential as therapeutic treatment for rheumatoid arthritis.[137]

BEWARE THE SWEET POTATO FRY

Of course, sweet potatoes have also been corrupted in much the same way as their more traditional friends and can now be found as sweet potato fries and chips. Since these sweet potatoes would be deep-fried in oil, their calorie content is typically substantially higher than the sweet potatoes you enjoy at home. You might also find sweet potato chips at the grocery or health food store, but once again, beware: Odds are they're packing about the same number of calories as an equal serving of French fries.

THE BOTTOM LINE

Sweet potatoes might not be superheroes when it comes to blood sugar, but it's hard to find a food higher in potassium or vitamin A anywhere. In many cases, putting sweet potatoes on your plate is nutritionally superior to a side of grains, especially grains that are white or refined—and, as luck would have it, they taste good, too.

WALNUTS

Just as almonds and avocados were banned from our diets during the low-fat diet craze, so were walnuts. It's taken a few decades to reha-bilitate their image, but walnuts, one of the two superstar tree nuts (along with almonds), are on everyone's superfood list. Of course, this can lead to a bit of healthy skepticism: Are walnuts really that good? Or are they just another overhyped superfood?

WALNUTS: THE STORY

Walnuts are a tree nut derived from the *Juglans regia* plant, which translates to "Jupiter's royal acorn." It was a common good traded on the Silk Road between Asia and the Middle East, and the term *English walnut* was coined when English merchants began transport-ing walnuts around the world—though, ironically, walnuts are not traditionally grown in England. Instead, they tend to flourish in Med-iterranean-like environments and are mentioned in various religious texts, including the Bible.

In California, where much of the walnut industry in the United States is based, walnuts are harvested from the end of August through November and are kept in whole form in cold storage for the rest of the year to keep the fats from oxidizing, or becoming rancid. Walnuts are usually available for purchase as halves or pieces, though in-shell walnuts that require cracking are also available. Since shelled walnuts are prone to becoming rancid, they should be eaten right away or else kept refrigerated. You can keep walnuts in the fridge for up to a month; any longer and they should be in the freezer.

WALNUTS: THE NUTRITION

A 1-ounce (28 gram) serving of walnuts, equal to approximately 14 halves of the edible part of the walnut (the hard shell should be discarded), provides 185 calories' worth of energy, along with 4 grams of protein and 2 grams of fibre. Although walnuts are particularly high in fat at 18 grams per serving, they are rich in omega-3 alpha-linolenic acid, or ALA, at 2.5 grams per serving, an amount that is on par with hemp seeds. The rest of their fat content is largely derived from omega-6 polyunsaturated fats (10.8 grams) and monounsaturated fats (2.5 grams).

Although walnuts are certainly nutritious, they don't fare as well as almonds when it comes to vitamins and minerals. They are a source of magnesium, providing 11% of your daily value, and are a good source of copper, at 22%, but they otherwise do not provide more than 10% of the daily value of any key nutrient. Although this makes walnuts seem a bit blah, their watershed moment came in 2006 when a study published in the *American Journal of Clinical Nutrition* found that walnuts had the highest antioxidant content of any common food, aside from a handful of herbs and spices.[138] When the antioxidant content was adjusted for typical serving sizes, walnuts finished second only to blackberries.

WALNUTS: THE SCIENCE
Walnuts and Heart Health

Although the fats and fibre in walnuts suggest they could have heart health benefits, the big reveal came in the spring of 2013 when the results of the PREDIMED study were published in the *New England Journal of Medicine*.[139] PREDIMED, which is short for the Spanish Prevención con Dieta Mediterránea (say it with me again . . . *Prevención con Dieta Mediterránea*. Nice.), is a rare long-term *prospective* dietary study, meaning that, instead of trying to get people to remember what they ate and hopefully linking it to disease risk after the fact, the researchers actually *put* the 7,500 participants on various dietary regimes and then watched what happened (the same was the case for the DASH diet study). At the start of the study, the subjects were randomly assigned to one of three Mediterranean-style diets: one with extra servings of olive oil, one with extra nuts (a combination of walnuts, almonds, and hazelnuts), or a low-fat diet that contained neither (control group). Although the subjects were asked to follow a Mediterranean diet, the food was not provided for them as it was in the DASH study, other than the appropriate daily servings of olive oil or nuts. After five years, the study was halted because the researchers felt the results were black and white: The olive oil and nut groups saw their risk of experiencing a cardiovascular event drop by an essentially equal 30% and 28% versus the "low-fat" group (note that the subjects in the low-fat group didn't really do their jobs very well and actually ended up eating some 37% of their calories from fat, much higher than the 30% recommendation, so it's probably better just to call that group the control group).

So, how much olive oil or nuts were the intervention groups eating? About 120 calories per day, which translates to about 1 tablespoon of olive oil or about 9 walnut halves per day—not much! Although, at first glance, this suggests that even a small addition of walnuts, almonds, hazelnuts, or olive oil to your diet can drastically alter your risk of disease, it's important to note that the intervention groups accidentally drifted in the healthy direction with their overall diets and ended up eating more fish and legumes, both of which also have known heart health benefits (now you see why the folks who ran the DASH diet were so scrupulous about what their subjects ate). So, whether walnuts are really that powerful for your heart remains to be seen, but for now, the results look promising.

But how do walnuts exert their effect? Cholesterol is one possibility. In a study on 21 men and women with high cholesterol, some of the same Spanish researchers placed subjects on either an olive oil–based Mediterranean diet or a diet rich in walnuts.[140] After four weeks, the walnut diet triggered a 4.4% drop in total cholesterol and a solid 6.4% drop in LDL cholesterol, and as with the PREDIMED study, the effect was statistically the same as the olive oil–based Mediterranean diet. In other words, when it comes to cholesterol control, walnuts may be just as effective as olive oil or other types of nuts. At least one study has even suggested that, for those genetically predisposed to high cholesterol, walnuts could even outdo olive oil when it comes to heart health.[141]

So, if we know that walnuts are a good choice for those at risk for heart attacks or strokes (like the people in the—say it with me one more time—Prevención con Dieta Mediterránea study), what about healthy people? That was the question on the minds of a group of researchers who examined the effect of eating about 1.5 to 2 ounces (or 21 to 28 halves) of walnuts per day, versus a walnut-free control diet, in 20 young Japanese men and women.[142] After four weeks on each diet, the walnut eaters had lower total cholesterol, and their ratio of LDL ("bad") to HDL ("good") cholesterol improved versus controls. The women—who, remember, were healthy to start the study—also saw a significant drop in their LDL cholesterol (the men didn't quite reach significance, which could be due to the relatively small size of the study group), and the walnut group also ended up with lower levels of apolipoprotein B, or apoB, the marker of small, dense LDL in the bloodstream.

As a source of omega-3 fatty acids (albeit in the less-potent plant form, ALA), walnuts might be assumed to have similar heart health benefits to fish. In reality, the effects of fish versus walnuts, while both seemingly good for our hearts, are actually very different. To wit: A 2009 study comparing the effects of daily consumption of 42 grams of walnuts (about 1.5 ounces) versus 4 ounces (113 grams) of salmon taken twice per week in 25 people with normal or slightly elevated cholesterol, found that the walnut eaters ended up with lower total and LDL cholesterol (not to mention apoB), while the fish eaters ended up with lower triglycerides and higher HDL.[143] The take-home message? Eat them both! Just make sure to keep portions of walnuts moderate: None of these studies used more than a handful or two per day.

Walnuts and Memory

If you surf the Web for long enough, odds are you'll eventually stumble across some site claiming that foods heal the part of the body they look like. Walnuts usually make this list because they look like a miniature brain. How cute! To some degree, these claims might actually have some validity, but as with blueberries, much of the research is in rats.[144] In the PREDIMED study, walnut consumption was associated with better working memory (remembering tasks, written lists, images, and so on) in older adults, though it didn't impact verbal memory (remembering instructions or conversations) or overall cognitive impairment.[145] In young adults, walnuts seem to have no effect on memory, mood, or non-verbal reasoning, though they may trigger a moderate improvement in inferential reasoning.[146] The bottom line? Although it's possible that nuts are good for our minds, we simply don't have enough data to say for sure, and the effects are probably small.

Walnuts and Weight Control

Despite the high calorie and high fat content of nuts, research has consistently demonstrated that nut consumption does not appear to be linked to weight gain or obesity; in fact, a number of studies have demonstrated that regular nut eaters tend to weigh less than those who don't eat nuts.[147] The fats in walnuts stimulate production of cholecystokinin, a protein that triggers feelings of fullness, and the fibre content could also play a role in appetite control. A handful of studies have demonstrated that eating walnuts before a meal (either at the previous meal or as part of a "preload" snack before a meal) results in increased feelings of fullness at the next meal.[148, 149] At the very least, walnuts, like all nuts, make a great choice for taking the edge off when you're about to hit a buffet, especially if you're famished: They might not fill you up, but they will at least give you a fighting chance at pushing the plate away before you've overdone it.

THE BOTTOM LINE

Walnuts taste good, are simple to eat, and have a lot of potential to help our hearts and our waistlines. Of course, as with all superfoods, sometimes the hype outpaces the evidence: Although walnuts do appear to be good for our hearts, their much-lauded impact on

cognitive function and memory is far from fact, and their antioxidant-rich status has yet to translate into any measurable health effect.
Otherwise, walnuts' appetite-suppressing effects could be useful for
weight control, though as with any calorie-rich foods, you still want
to keep an eye on your portions: A handful a day is probably enough.

5

SEND ME A HERO

OVERLOOKED AND UNDERAPPRECIATED SUPERFOODS

Okay, so spinach is good for you. And so are walnuts. No surprise there, and if you're reading this book, there's a good chance those are already on your grocery list. But does that mean we're at the end of the road for high-nutrient foods that are readily available in North America? Definitely not. There are still plenty of under-the-radar foods that have their own stories to tell. When was the last time you ate collard greens? And why go out of your way to eat sesame seeds or mussels? Let's wrap up this discussion with a section dedicated to superfoods that tend to get passed by but deserve a bit more of our attention.

AMARANTH

Unless you've been living under a rock, you've probably at least heard of quinoa, and you might have even tried it. But what about amaranth? With a similar nutrition profile, this pseudograin seems to have almost as much to offer our diets as its South American cousin, yet it has received far less attention in North America.

AMARANTH: THE STORY

Although often prepared and used as a grain, amaranth is actually a seed derived from a tall, broad-leafed plant that is part of the Amaranthaceae family. Since it is not a member of the Poaceae family, from which true cereal grains (such as oats and wheat) are derived, amaranth, much like quinoa, is considered a pseudograin or pseudocereal. A staple in Central and South America for some 6,000 to 8,000 years, amaranth made its way to Asia as contraband in the 16th century when Cortez and the Spanish conquistadores banned its cultivation as a means of destroying the Aztecs.

AMARANTH: THE NUTRITION

A cup of cooked amaranth has a nutrition profile similar to quinoa, providing 251 calories, 9 grams of protein (quinoa has 8 grams), and an equal 5 grams of fibre. Impressively, a cup of amaranth provides 5 mg of iron, or just under 30% of your daily needs, twice the amount in a comparable serving of quinoa. Unfortunately, like many plant foods, amaranth contains compounds known as phytates that limit our ability to absorb the iron it contains. In fact, research on iron-deficient and anemic Kenyan preschoolers found that consuming an iron-fortified porridge helped improve their iron status, but an amaranth-based porridge did not.[1]

Amaranth is also known for being far more calcium-rich than quinoa, offering up 12% of your daily requirements, or 116 mg, per cup, while quinoa provides a mere 3%. It is also higher in magnesium, providing 40% of your daily needs (versus 30% for quinoa). Amaranth has about the same amount of potassium as a banana and offers 10% of your daily requirements of zinc, copper, and selenium. It is slightly less rich in B vitamins than quinoa and is also lower in vitamin E, but it is still a good source of vitamin B$_6$ and folate. All in all, if quinoa is among the kings of all superfoods, amaranth should at least be its queen. Since amaranth is only now emerging on the North American market, however, we don't have complete nutrition information: The USDA database, for example, does not yet include its full amino acid profile.

Like quinoa, amaranth is gluten free, and it is another grain that provides the complete array of essential amino acids, including lysine, an amino acid that is uncommon to many plant foods. One potential drawback of amaranth, however, is that it seems to have a high glycemic index (GI), meaning it could trigger a rapid rise in blood sugar.[2] The relatively small starch granules inside amaranth seeds may be responsible for this unexpected phenomenon (starches, also known as complex carbohydrates, tend to exist as granules inside a food; larger granules are usually slower to break down, causing a more gradual rise in blood sugar, while smaller granules break down more quickly). Indeed, studies examining the blood sugar effects of flatbreads made with mixtures of amaranth and wheat flour suggest that the more amaranth flour the bread contains (versus wheat flour), the higher the GI climbs. Also, studies on popped amaranth, mixed with milk and an artificial sweetener (milk is generally low GI, and the artificial sweetener shouldn't have any effect on blood sugar) have found it to have a startlingly high GI of 97, just a step below the GI of 100 for pure glucose. This is early data, however, and we need more research on the blood sugar effects of amaranth in mixed meals before we toss out this otherwise nutrient-rich grain.

AMARANTH: THE SCIENCE

Studies on chickens (yes, chickens), hamsters, and rats suggest that amaranth and amaranth oil could have potential cholesterol- and triglyceride-lowering effects.[3, 4, 5] Amaranth is also said to possess immune-system-modulating effects and antitumour activity, as well as being rich in antioxidants, including being a relatively rare source (aside from fish) of the natural skin moisturizer squalene.[6] Unfortunately, our knowledge of the benefits of amaranth and amaranth oil largely ends there; to date, there are no well-controlled human studies examining amaranth's effects on health or disease.

EATING AMARANTH

Like other grains and pseudograins, amaranth can be cooked by simmering for about 20 minutes in water or stock until tender. Generally, a ratio of two-and-a-half to three parts water or broth is used for every one part of uncooked amaranth (use smaller amounts of water for pilafs and savoury dishes, or larger amounts to make a porridge). Popped amaranth is also popular as a snack; simply place the dry amaranth in a pot or pan on high heat and stir. Once the seeds have popped, remove them and add more (avoid overcrowding the pan). Amaranth flour can also be used in baking, most commonly making up to a quarter of the total flour content in gluten-containing or gluten-free recipes.

THE BOTTOM LINE

With so much pressure on our global food system, amaranth has good potential to serve as a nutritious alternative to our staple foods, including rice, corn, and wheat. Known for its high yield, hardiness, and tolerance of dry conditions, amaranth can be grown in what would traditionally be viewed as poor conditions. As a result, researchers and agricultural experts are increasingly recommending its adoption into our food system, with a particular focus on its ability to support improved nutrition in developing countries.

COLLARD GREENS

Like the bridesmaid who is never the bride, collard greens don't receive nearly the level of popular attention that kale has been afforded in recent years, yet they are just as worthy of the public's affection as their equally green cousin.

COLLARD GREENS: THE STORY

Collard greens, originally known as colewort, are a part of the cabbage, or *Brassica*, family. Collards and kale are so closely related that they actually share the same botanical name, *Brassica oleracea*, variety *acephala*—also known as the headless cabbage group (somehow, this seems to evoke images of a cabbage riding through a dark forest, but I didn't get the feeling that the collards I have eaten were on a quest for vengeance). The only difference between the two is in the styling of the leaves: Collard greens are wider and flatter, while kale tends to have a curly, frilled appearance.

Collard greens have a long history of use in the U.S. South, where they are commonly consumed on New Year's Day as a means of attracting wealth. In fact, collard greens are the second-most popular food—not just vegetable—of any kind among older adults living in the U.S. South.[7]

The peak season for collard greens is from January to April, though they can usually be found in grocery stores year-round. Preference for collard greens might, at least in part, be dictated by genetics.[8] The high calcium content might also add a certain bitterness that makes them less palatable for some.[9]

Collard greens can be enjoyed in a variety of ways, including stir-fried and steamed (just wash and slice or chop the collards into 1- to 2-inch chunks before cooking), but if you want true southern eating, then preparing collards with black-eyed peas and shrimp or as a gumbo is the way to go.

COLLARD GREENS: THE NUTRITION

Put simply, collard greens are profoundly nutritious. A cup of chopped collard greens, boiled from frozen, provides 5 grams each of fibre and protein, along with just 61 calories. Now comes the fun: You'll also pick up 391% of your vitamin A, 75% of your vitamin C, and 1,324% of your vitamin K (no, that's not a typo) needs for a day. Add to that 32% of your folate and 36% of your calcium—that's more than you'll get from a glass of milk—and you'll see why it's easy to get excited about this emerald-hued veggie (collards do contain oxalates, however, which likely impedes our ability to absorb at least some of the calcium, though no one, to date, has determined just how much[10]). As if that's not enough, you'll also pick up at least 10% of your vitamins B_2, B_6, and E, as well as the minerals iron, magnesium, and potassium. Like kale, collard greens are rich in other compounds that may have disease-fighting properties, known as phenolics, including kaempferol, quercetin, and a family of compounds known as glucosinolates.[11]

COLLARD GREENS: THE SCIENCE

There is evidence that both kale and collard greens may be protective against glaucoma. In a 2012 study published in the *American Journal of Ophthalmology*, UCLA researchers found that, among 662 older African-American women, those who consumed at least one serving of kale and collard greens per month had a 57% lower chance of developing glaucoma versus those who consumed them less than once per month.[12] An earlier study on women of various ethnicities found a similar result.[13]

There is also evidence to suggest that collard greens, along with kale and mustard greens, have cholesterol-lowering capacity, at least in part by binding bile salts, which naturally contain cholesterol, in the digestive tract, causing them to be excreted in our feces. In one study, steamed (but not raw) collards seemed to be as effective for cholesterol control as the drug cholestyramine (Questran), which also lowers cholesterol by removing bile salts from the body.[14] Aside from bile acid sequestering, the glucosinolates found in collard greens also seem to have anti-inflammatory effects that could be protective against heart disease; this theory, however, requires more research to be validated.

Also, consuming a diet rich in *Brassica* vegetables, including broccoli, cabbage, mustard greens, and collard greens, as well as bok choy, may be protective against numerous other types of cancer, including prostate cancer[15] and stomach, esophageal (gastric), and lung cancers.[16] Part of the effect might be attributable to the carotenoids, or vitamin A, in dark green vegetables, which have been inconsistently linked to cancer prevention. Why the uncertainty about whether or not carotenoids, like beta-carotene, are cancer fighters? It might be that we haven't been looking in the right place: Most studies try to link carotenes in our diets to cancer risk, but a 2012 study suggested that the amount of carotenoids actually circulating in our blood could be the better predictor of our risk of developing cancer.[17] While researchers work to better understand the role diet can play in cancer prevention, your best bet is to include dark red, orange, and green veggies (which, collectively, are the richest sources of carotenoids) in your diet on a regular basis.

THE BOTTOM LINE

In a world where we are constantly bombarded with the latest trends in diet and nutrition, somehow collard greens have remained under the radar. Yet with a nutrition profile no less impressive than kale's and the potential to control cholesterol, fight cancer, and prevent debilitating conditions such as macular degeneration, collards deserve a spot on almost any superfood list.

KIWI FRUIT

With its tough, brown exterior, kiwi fruit, often shortened to kiwi, doesn't always seem worth the bother. How, exactly, do you remove the skin without mangling the fruit and leaving yourself covered in mushy, green pulp? These issues, plus kiwi's still-exotic vibe (despite the fact that California is now one of the world's leading kiwi producers), seem to leave kiwis on the sidelines when it comes to lunchbags: As of 2009, the average Canadian consumed about four kiwis per year.[18] But make no mistake: Kiwis are nutritional heavyweights that have been vastly underappreciated.

KIWI FRUIT: THE STORY

Kiwi fruit was first cultivated in China, where it was considered a delicacy and was used for medicinal treatment of conditions related to pain and inflammation, including gout and rheumatoid arthritis. Known scientifically as *Actinidia polygama*, kiwi fruit eventually migrated southward to New Zealand, where it earned the nickname Chinese gooseberry. According to legend, the first kiwis were imported to the United States in the 1960s for a lone shopper at a Safeway grocery store in California who requested the fruit from a produce clerk. So, how did it end up with the kiwi name? After the equally fuzzy brown bird from New Zealand, of course.

In California, kiwis are harvested from October to May, and in Chile and New Zealand, they are harvested in what is spring and summer in the northern hemisphere. Translation? They are available year-round in many grocery stores. When buying kiwi fruit, look for fruit that has intact, unblemished skin; when pressed, the fruit should give slightly. If it is too firm, it isn't ready to eat, and if it is very soft and wrinkled, it is overripe. Kiwi fruit will ripen in a few days if left at room temperature, or you can store them in the fridge for several weeks. If you are trying to encourage your kiwi fruit to ripen a bit faster, try storing them alongside an apple or banana in a plastic bag (just be sure to allow a slight opening) for a day or two.

Kiwi fruit can be eaten in its entirety, skin and all—just be sure to give it a good rinse if you plan to eat the skin—otherwise, you can trim off the skin and eat the interior "meat" of the fruit any way you like. One final option is to "sloop" the kiwi, a term coined by California Kiwifruit, which means to slice the fruit in half, lengthwise, and then use a spoon to scoop the meat away from the flesh.[19] Kiwis may be best enjoyed raw, but they also make great additions to fruit salads, desserts, lemonade, and smoothies.

KIWI FRUIT: THE NUTRITION

A cup of kiwi (177 grams), which translates to about 2 large kiwis (91 grams each), *without the skin*, provides 108 calories' worth of energy, along with 5 grams of fibre and 16 grams of sugar. When it comes to vitamin C, kiwi towers over the competition: A cup of kiwi provides 273% of your daily needs, more than twice the amount in an equal serving of oranges!

Kiwis are also exceptionally high in vitamin K, providing 89% of your daily needs per cup; are a rare fruit that is a good source of vitamin E (13% of your daily requirements per cup); and are a source of vitamin B_6, folate, calcium, magnesium, potassium, and copper. Kiwi is also one of the richest food sources of lutein, a carotenoid (member of the vitamin A family) that makes up part of the retina of our eyes and is thought to guard against age-related macular degeneration.[20]

KIWI FRUIT: THE SCIENCE
Kiwi Fruit and Heart Health

In 2004, a pair of Norwegian researchers published a study that examined the effect on healthy volunteers of consuming two or three kiwi fruit per day for 28 days.[21] At the end of the study period, the subjects' serum (blood) levels of triglycerides, the fats that make up part of the cholesterol profile, dropped by 15%, a result that is particularly impressive when you consider that eating sugar (kiwi, like all fruit, naturally contains a modest amount of sugar) tends to make triglycerides go up, not down. The subjects also saw a decline in markers of platelet aggregation, which is thought to play a role in the development of plaques in our arteries that can eventually lead to heart attacks and strokes. In a similar study on 43 men and women with high cholesterol, those who ate two kiwis per day saw their HDL cholesterol levels rise significantly from the start of the study.[22] Unfortunately, both studies did not include control groups (a comparable group of individuals who did not consume kiwi during the study), which means they are considered a lower quality of research, and the results need to be verified in better-controlled studies.

A study that did include controls, published in 2012 by New Zealand researchers, demonstrated that adding two kiwi fruit per day for four weeks to the diet of 85 men with elevated cholesterol levels caused a small but significant increase in HDL ("good") cholesterol as well as a drop in triglycerides in individuals with a certain genetic subtype that makes them more susceptible to heart disease and

Alzheimer's, known as the APOE4 allele.[23] Total cholesterol, LDL cholesterol, blood pressure, blood glucose, insulin, and C-reactive protein, a measure of inflammation in the body, were unchanged. The study was a crossover study by design, which means the subjects acted as their own controls by also following a four-week diet period without any kiwi, making it stronger than the Norwegian study and suggesting that a normal "dose" of just two kiwis per day may have some benefit on heart health markers within a month or less.

Kiwi Fruit and Cancer Prevention

Kiwi fruit has been studied for its antioxidant value as well as for its potential for cancer prevention. A study conducted using the less-common golden kiwi fruit, *Actinidia chinensis*, found that giving one or two kiwi fruit per day to healthy adults increased circulating levels of vitamin C and resulted in reduced oxidative DNA damage to lymphocyte (white blood) cells.[24] Other cell line studies have also found that kiwi fruit extract can protect against DNA damage, even more so than a comparable dose of vitamin C.[25] Although these results suggest that kiwi fruit could protect against DNA damage, research has yet to clearly link either DNA damage or oxidative damage in *in vitro* studies such as these to a lower risk of developing cancer in real-life situations. Nonetheless, as with many fruits and vegetables, the available data we have suggests that kiwi fruit might well help have some effect on cancer prevention.

Kiwi Fruit for the Bowel

With 5 grams of fibre per two-fruit serving, it makes sense that kiwi fruit could keep the plumbing moving, and, as luck would have it, a research team from Taipei confirmed this assumption. In their study, 54 adults with irritable bowel syndrome (IBS), a medical condition characterized by abdominal pain, diarrhea, and constipation, were given two kiwi fruit per day for four weeks. At the end of the trial, the subjects, all of whom were characterized as having IBS with constipation, had significantly more bowel movements, and colon transit time (the amount of time it takes for food to travel through the digestive system) decreased; in other words, kiwi seemed to help "get things moving," which would no doubt bring welcome relief for those suffering from constipation.[26] Studies on elderly populations have also found that kiwi fruit can improve bowel health and can help reduce reliance on commercial laxatives.[27, 28] These studies suggest that kiwi can do a bowel—even an irritable one—some good.

Kiwi Fruit and the Skin

With its high concentration of vitamin C, it would be expected that kiwi fruit could help to improve or maintain skin health by promoting the production of collagen, a compound known for its importance to skin elasticity. Although good-quality research on the effects of food on skin health are rare, at least one cell line study demonstrated that sugars from the kiwi fruit doubled the production of collagen in human skin cells and skin equivalents.[29]

THE BOTTOM LINE

Despite their fabulous value, kiwis still seem like a delicacy rather than a mainstay. Surprisingly easy to eat (once you figure out how to sloop, you're laughing), kiwis contain more vitamin C than an orange and more potassium than a banana, and yet Canadians eat only a fraction of the amount they consume of their more commonplace counterparts. So, next time you are looking for an easy fruit to toss in your lunch, to perk up a smoothie, or as part of a fruit salad, consider the fuzzy brown fruit named for a foreign bird.

OYSTERS AND MUSSELS

Yes, yes, we know: Salmon is good for you. It's been done to death, and in some ways, it could be the death of us. After all, salmon farms have been heavily criticized for their environmental track record, which has included the accidental release of harmful lice and diseases into the oceans when the occasional salmon escapes from its pen. As a predatory fish, salmon also cost the environment in other ways, by requiring other fish to be harvested to produce their meal or by eating other fish when they are in the wild, reducing other fish populations. Although salmon remains perhaps the best choice for omega-3 fatty acids, that doesn't mean it is the only option, and others can be gentler on our planet. Looking for a recommendation? How about giving oysters and mussels a try?

OYSTERS AND MUSSELS: THE STORY

Oysters and mussels are technically bivalve molluscs. When oysters are invaded by a parasite, they cover it with a protective layer, known as a nacre. If left for a few years, that nacre will eventually lead to the formation of a pearl. Oysters are decidedly lower on the evolutionary scale than many fish and fowl—in some cases they are considered acceptable food for vegans because they lack a central nervous system, but they do possess a small heart and even two kidneys. Mussels can be enjoyed either inside or out of their long, thin shell, often in a light tomato sauce. Or they can be prepared as muurugai as part of sushi.

OYSTERS AND MUSSELS: THE NUTRITION

While oysters may be seen as a delicacy, their nutritional value makes you wish they could be a staple food: 3 ounces (85 grams) of farmed Eastern oysters, equivalent to about eight medium, provides 6 grams of protein along with just 2 grams of fat, of which 179 mg is DHA and 195 mg is EPA. Although those numbers are low compared with oily fish, which can provide more than 1000 mg of EPA and DHA per serving, remember that eight oysters contain a paltry 67 calories, far less than the 250 or so calories in a salmon filet.

Outside of their macronutrients (meaning the protein, carbohydrates, and fats they contain), oysters are also impressively rich in numerous vitamins and minerals: They offer not only a remarkable 6.6 mg of iron, or about 37% of an average adult's needs for a day (a comparable serving of beef, by comparison, offers up 2 mg), but also 61% of your copper and 94% of your selenium for the day. But that's not even the most impressive part: You'll also pick up 256%—yes, two-and-a-half days' worth—of your zinc requirements and 344%, or half a week's worth, of vitamin B_{12}, an important vitamin for the development of healthy red blood cells. While those are the headliners for the nutrients from oysters. They also provide at least 5% of your daily needs for vitamin C, thiamin (vitamin B_1), niacin (vitamin B_3), folate, calcium, and magnesium.

Far more protein-rich, a 3-ounce (85 gram) serving of cooked blue mussels provides 20 grams of muscle-building protein, a fairly modest 146 calories, and 4 grams of fat, of which 430 mg are from DHA and 235 mg from EPA (by comparison, the American Heart Association recommends two servings of oily fish per week, translating into roughly 500 mg of EPA and DHA, the two omega-3 fats found mostly in fish and in smaller amounts in some forms of algae and in mammals raised on grass or pasture, per day), so you're getting more than a day's worth of omega-3 from just a handful of the dark-shelled delicacy.

Like oysters, however, the beauty of mussels is far deeper than the protein and fat content. They also provide 19% of your vitamin C (interesting, since we don't tend to associate vitamin C with animal foods), 17% of your vitamin B_1, 21% of your vitamin B_2, 13% of your niacin vitamin B_3, and 16% of your folate (another nutrient that tends to be associated with plants, not animal foods). But the clincher, in terms of vitamins, is vitamin B_{12}, a nutrient often associated with deficiency in older adults: 340% of your daily needs.

Vitamins aside, mussels are also a source of numerous minerals, including 32% of your iron and 15% of your zinc. Like many types of seafood, they are also incredibly high in selenium: 3 ounces provides 109% of your daily needs. They also offer almost three days' worth of manganese, a mineral that generally isn't an issue when it comes to deficiency but an impressive number nonetheless. They are also a source of vitamin A (5%), magnesium (8%), potassium (7%, or 228 mg), and copper (6%). In other words, mussels are a source of almost every major and minor nutrient the human body needs.

OYSTERS AND MUSSELS: THE SCIENCE

Diets rich in shellfish have often been thought to have negative effects on our heart health because of their relatively high cholesterol content. In truth, however, shellfish, including both oysters and mussels, seem to have heart health benefits. In a 1990 study, published in the *American Journal of Clinical Nutrition*, 18 men with normal lipid levels were fed various shellfish, including oysters, mussels, clams, crabs, squid, and shrimp.[30] At the end of the study, mussels and oysters lowered triglycerides and raised HDL cholesterol, and both were also associated with a better ratio of LDL to HDL ("bad" to "good") cholesterol. Although mussels did not have a statistically significant effect on LDL cholesterol, oysters did. By comparison, clams and crabs had lesser effects on cholesterol, and shrimp and squid demonstrated no benefit at all. An earlier study by the same research team found that our bodies seem to absorb less cholesterol from oysters than from chicken and crab.[31] A study on the effects of low-carbohydrate diets (either rich in red meats or poultry, fish, and shellfish), conducted in moderately obese subjects, found that diets rich in shellfish had an equal effect on weight loss as a red meat diet, along with a more pronounced effect on triglycerides, a result that is not surprising when you consider that a high intake of omega-3 fatty acids is a known treatment for elevated triglycerides.[32]

CONSEQUENCES OF CONSUMPTION

The depletion of fish stocks is a serious ecological issue the world over, and our increased emphasis on omega-3 fat has been part of the problem: According to experts in the area, the extraction of omega-3 fatty acids from fish is a serious environmental concern. As filter feeders, however, oysters and mussels actually filter the ocean, taking water in across their gills and trapping small particles such as plankton in the process. It's for this reason that Monterey Bay Aquarium's renowned Seafood Watch gave several varieties of oysters, including wild and farmed American, Blue Points Common, Eastern, and Kaki oysters, a Best Choice rating.[33] Monterey Bay also gives the thumbs up to farming—also known as aquaculture—of mussels, as they rarely require antibiotics, and farming can be conducted in an environmentally sound way.[34] In particular, blue, black, and green mussels from all over the world were given the Best Choice recommendation.

THE BOTTOM LINE

When it comes to fish and shellfish, it's easy to feel guilty. Although both are wildly nutritious, with global fish stocks under enormous strain, it seems there is rarely good news. Bearing in mind both environmental and nutritional concerns, it is reassuring to know that oysters and mussels can be good for us, and for the planet.

PISTACHIOS

If you follow nutrition in the media, odds are you've heard that almonds and walnuts are good for you. The love affair with these two nuts runs so deep you might be left with the impression they are the only two nuts in existence. So unfair! In reality, there are so many other nuts out there pining for a little attention. Among the sick-of-being-forgotten tree nuts is the pistachio, the once-red nut with the clam-style shell that has more to offer than just being a popular ice cream flavour. So, for the poor pistachios' sake, please give them a second look.

PISTACHIOS: THE STORY

Pistachios are the nuts of the flowering *Pistacia vera* plant and are derived from the same family (Anacardiaceae) as the cashew. Pistachio plants are believed to have originated in Iran, and the nuts have a long history of human use, dating back some 9,000 years. Historically speaking, pistachios are one of two nuts mentioned in the Bible and are said to have been found in the hanging gardens of Babylon. For years, they were used as an energy source during prolonged travel and were commonly eaten by traders travelling along the Silk Road from China to the West. According to legend, the Queen of Sheba was so enamoured with pistachios that she decreed her entire region's crop be devoted just to her.[35]

Today, pistachios are cultivated in warm climates, including Afghanistan and the Mediterranean. In the United States, pistachios are grown almost exclusively in California, where they have been cultivated since the 1970s. For years, pistachios were dyed red, partly to hide their imperfections and partly to attract more consumer attention.

Pistachios grow in clusters, much like grapes. In the late summer and early fall, they ripen, causing the hard exterior shell to split. Even though the shell has split, however, pistachio fans still bear the responsibility of breaking them fully open to get at the kernel inside. Although this is usually a relatively easy process, from time to time you might encounter a devilishly difficult nut to crack. If that's the case, the good folks at instructables.com recommend wedging the shell from a previously enjoyed nut into the partially opened pistachio and then twisting it like a screwdriver.[36] On the other hand, if the shell is completely closed, then it means the pistachio is not ripe and should be discarded. This open style of shell among ripened pistachios is presumably the genesis of the term "smiling nut" or "happy nut" used to describe pistachios in Iran and China.

PISTACHIOS: THE NUTRITION

For all the attention afforded to almonds and walnuts, it might surprise you to see just how well pistachios compare. An ounce (28 grams) of pistachios (about 49 kernels) provides 157 calories' worth of energy, along with the same amount of protein (6 grams) and fibre (3 grams) as an equal serving of almonds. Overall, pistachios are the richest of the three in B vitamins, especially B_1 (16% of your daily needs) and B_6 (24%). They are also the highest in iron (7%), albeit marginally so, while also providing 9% of your magnesium and 290 mg of potassium, or 8% of your daily value.

In terms of fats, pistachios are particularly rich in monounsaturated fats, or MUFAs, providing about 7 grams per serving. Their omega-3 fatty acid content is low, however, especially in relation to their omega-6 content (72 mg versus 3,729 mg); with evidence that humans evolved with omega-3 to omega-6 ratios of roughly 1:4 or less, and with current estimates that our intake skews much more heavily toward omega-6s, there is a popular notion that we should be eating less omega-6 and more omega-3. This theory, though, still needs more research, and for now, Health Canada continues to recommend consuming omega-6 fats, especially in lieu of saturated fats or trans fats. Major nutrients aside, pistachio nuts are also higher in nutrients with potential antioxidant and disease-fighting properties, including lutein, beta-carotene, and a type of vitamin E known as gamma-tocopherol, compared with other nuts.

PISTACHIOS: THE SCIENCE

Pistachios and Heart Health

To date, five randomized trials have examined the effects of pistachios on levels of cholesterol and triglycerides, collectively known as lipids. In 2008, researchers from Pennsylvania State University, one of the top nutrition schools in the United States, published a randomized crossover study examining the effects of one or two servings of pistachios per day on 28 adults with high cholesterol.[37] At the start of the study, much like the DASH diet study, participants were placed on a traditional Western diet for two weeks (remember, this helps ensure that

COMPARING SOME COMMON NUTRIENTS IN THREE DIFFERENT NUTS

ITEM	Almonds	Walnuts	Pistachios
AMOUNT	1 ounce (28 g) = 23 kernels	1 ounce (28 g) = 14 halves	1 ounce (28 g) = 49 kernels
Calories	162	185	157
Fat	14 g	14 g	13 g
Carbohydrate	6 g	4 g	8 g
Fibre	3 g	2 g	3 g
Protein	6 g	5 g	6 g
Vitamin E	37%	1%	3%
Vitamin B_1	4%	6%	16%
Vitamin B_2	17%	2%	3%
Vitamin B_3	5%	2%	2%
Vitamin B_6	2%	8%	24%
Folate	4%	7%	4%
Calcium	7%	3%	3%
Iron	6%	5%	7%
Magnesium	19%	11%	9%
Phosphorus	14%	10%	14%
Potassium	6%	4%	8%
Zinc	6%	6%	4%
Copper	14%	22%	18%
Selenium	1%	2%	3%

Source: USDA National Nutrient Database

everyone has a similar starting point). Thereafter, subjects were fed a diet with either zero, one, or two servings of pistachios per day (the size of the serving varied with the participants' energy needs, but the amount ranged from about 1 to 2 ounces per day for the one-serving group and about 2 to 4 ounces per day for the two-serving group). Throughout the study, the subjects kept their caloric intake steady so that any effect observed could be isolated to the pistachios, not weight loss.

At the end of the study (subjects completed four weeks on each diet in random order), there was a clear dose-dependent effect of pistachios on cholesterol and other associated risk factors for heart disease. For example, the high-dose group saw their total cholesterol drop by 8%, their LDL cholesterol by 12%, and their non-HDL cholesterol (all the types of cholesterol except the "good" HDL) by 11%. In addition, their levels of apolipoprotein B (apoB), the marker of small, dense LDL—considered the most harmful type of LDL— dropped by 4%. In comparison, the single-dose group saw their cholesterol levels improve, but not quite as much: For example, their LDL dropped by only 3% versus 12% in the two-dose group. Several other clinical trials have produced similar outcomes as the Penn State study, suggesting that a dose of 2 to 3 ounces of pistachios per day can have a significant effect on cholesterol, with the most consistent effect being an increase in HDL.[38, 39, 40]

Pistachios and Weight Control

Aside from their effect on cholesterol, it has been speculated that pistachios, along with other nuts, can help us control our weight, and a few studies have investigated this hypothesis. In 2010, a group of researchers published a study examining the effects of eating pistachios instead of pretzels (a high-carbohydrate food that is low in fibre, healthy fats, and protein—basically, the opposite of pistachios) on weight loss in a group of 59 obese adults.[41] As part of the study, participants were placed on a weight-loss diet, but they were given different (but roughly equal-calorie) afternoon snacks: 240 calories (53 grams) of salted pistachios or 220 calories (26 grams) of salted pretzels. At the end of the 12-week study, both groups lost weight, but the pistachio group lost significantly more than the pretzel group and also finished with lower triglycerides. This provides evidence for what many have already suggested, namely that protein, fibre, and foods rich in healthy fats, such as pistachios, may be better for our waistlines than refined carbohydrate, and it confirms previous findings that refined carbohydrate foods do naughty things to our triglyceride levels.

Although nuts may be associated with healthy weight control, the effect they have is probably slight, and perhaps non-existent, depending on the rest of your diet's makeup. Case in point: Chinese researchers recently gave a group of 90 patients with metabolic syndrome (the cluster of conditions associated with an increased risk of cardiovascular disease and type 2 diabetes) moderate (42 g/day, or about 1.5 ounces) or high (70 g/day, or about 2.5 ounces) doses of pistachios, or no pistachios at all, each day for 12 weeks.[42] Otherwise, the subjects did not change their usual diets. At the end of the study, the pistachio eaters' weight was unchanged, and their waist-to-hip ratio (a measure of body fat around the abdomen, considered the most dangerous type of fat) was no different from the pistachio-avoiding controls. In other words, pistachios and other nuts might be good for you and could have appetite-suppressing effects, but if you do add them to your diet, it needs to be in exchange for something else (preferably less nutritious, such as pretzels, bagels, granola bars, or sweets), rather than just noshing on nuts and hoping the weight will just magically fall off.

Pistachios and Glycemic Control

In a small study conducted by Dr. David Jenkins' group at St. Michael's Hospital and the University of Toronto, 10 otherwise healthy overweight adults were given 1, 2, or 3 ounces of pistachios in a meal with white bread to see just how much the pistachios could lessen the blood-sugar-raising effect of eating white bread and other carbohydrate-containing foods alone.[43] As expected, eating pistachios blunted the blood sugar response from the bread, reducing it by 11%, 33%, and 48% for the 1-, 2-, and 3-ounce servings, respectively, and also reduced the blood sugar effect of eating parboiled rice and pasta (both carbohydrate-based foods that would turn into sugar fairly quickly). Although these results suggest that adding pistachios—and presumably other nuts—to a carbohydrate-containing meal can help keep blood sugars from spiking, remember that you add about 160 calories for each ounce of pistachios you consume with your meal; as a result, your best bet is to cut down on the portions of starches and then complement with moderate portions of pistachios or other protein- and fibre-rich foods.

Pistachios and Erectile Dysfunction

In a 2011 study, Turkish researchers found that giving men 100 grams of pistachios per day for three weeks resulted in improved sexual function (assessed via the International Index of Erectile Function, which improved by an average of 50% from the start of the study) as well as improved total, LDL, and HDL cholesterol levels. Unfortunately, the lack of a control arm in the study means some of the effect could have been a placebo response or due to other changes to their diets during the study. It should also be noted that the dose of pistachios (about 3.5 ounces per day, or about 550 calories' worth) was very high. Clearly, more research is needed, but this study follows the same line of logic we have seen from other studies: that a heart-healthy diet may exert effects on the vascular system throughout our bodies, not just in our hearts.

THE BOTTOM LINE

Although almonds and walnuts have enjoyed well-deserved time in the spotlight, it's time to pass the torch on to other nuts, and pistachios are a worthy heir apparent. With good evidence that they can improve measures of heart health, especially HDL ("good") cholesterol, pistachios may have benefits that extend well beyond our hearts. And one added benefit: Those hard shells will slow you down, which should keep you from overdoing it. Otherwise, enjoy!

PUMPKIN SEEDS

Often relegated to the post-Halloween garbage bin, pumpkin seeds, also known as pepitas, have enjoyed a minor resurgence in popularity in recent years, and for good reason. They still, however, remain a fringe food that is all-too-easily forgotten among the almonds, walnuts, hemp, and chia seeds of the world.

PUMPKIN SEEDS: THE STORY

Pumpkins are the fruit of *Cucurbita* plants and are a member of the Cucurbitaceae, or gourd, family, which also includes melons and squash. An unusually large fruit, pumpkins are usually between 9 and 18 pounds but in extremes can grow up to 75 pounds. Common to North America and Europe, pumpkin is often eaten as a side dish (which itself is very nutritious). The pumpkin's seeds have a cream-coloured hull, with the olive green seeds found inside. Slightly larger and flatter than sesame seeds, pumpkin seeds are mild tasting and easier to chew than many nuts.

Pumpkin seeds can be eaten raw or roasted, in the shell or hulled. You can add pumpkin seeds to salads or trail mixes (they pair particularly well with dried cranberries and ginger), and they can be sprinkled on baked goods, including breads and muffins. Pumpkin seed oil can be used as a salad dressing, though its low smoke point means it is not typically recommended for cooking or frying. Since they don't need to be refrigerated, pumpkin seeds are great for travelling and can be transported in school bags and left in desk drawers for a week or two, where they make a great choice for an afternoon snack.

PUMPKIN SEEDS: THE NUTRITION

Perhaps the most significant of pumpkin seeds' claims to fame centres on their iron content: A 1-ounce (28 gram) serving of pumpkin seed kernels (the softer part of the seed found inside the tougher shell) provides about 23% of our daily iron needs, making them, along with pulses, some of the richest non-meat sources of iron available. Pumpkin seeds are also a good source of protein, providing 9 grams per ounce, which is more than you'll find in an egg or a glass of milk, although it does not contain all the essential amino acids that serve as the building blocks of protein, making pumpkin seeds a lower-quality protein source than animal foods.

Pumpkin seeds are also one of the best food sources of magnesium, the often underappreciated mineral that plays a role in blood pressure control, bone health, and muscle function. Magnesium's muscle-relaxing effects may help with constipation as well as ease the restless, achy legs that are common in athletes and older adults, especially those taking statin (cholesterol) drugs. Higher magnesium intakes have also been associated with a lower risk of both stroke and colorectal cancer. Unfortunately, many North Americans do not meet their daily requirements (320 mg per day for women, 420 mg per day for men), in large part since magnesium-rich foods, such as fish, nuts, seeds, and green leafy vegetables, are not always the most popular foods. Since a 1-ounce serving of pumpkin seeds provides an impressive 151 mg of magnesium, equivalent to 36% of an adult male's needs, they make an easy choice to help meet the requirements of this important yet underconsumed nutrient.

Like all nuts and seeds, pumpkin seeds are relatively high in calories, so portion control is important: That same 1-ounce serving packs 146 calories, and if you were to enjoy a full 1-cup serving, you would put away more than 1,100 calories' worth of energy, more than a half-day's worth for most adults!

PUMPKIN SEEDS: THE SCIENCE

Like soybeans, pumpkin seeds contain phytoestrogens, compounds that mimic estrogen in the human body. As a result, there is a question as to whether or not pumpkin seeds can influence the risk of certain hormone-dependent cancers, especially breast cancer. Although the research on pumpkin seeds in humans is limited, a 2012 study on nearly 3,000 post-menopausal German women, published in the journal *Nutrition and Cancer*, found that regular consumption of soybeans, sunflower seeds, and pumpkin seeds was associated with a reduced risk of breast cancer versus controls.[44] There are also suggestions that pumpkin seed oil may have heart health benefits.[45]

As for the high iron content of pumpkin seeds, since they are a plant food, it is possible that only a limited amount of the iron is actually available for use by the body, yet since iron-deficiency anemia is an enormously burdensome health-care issue, especially in the developing world, there is great interest in finding foods that are cost effective and can have a significant effect on iron status. To test the effect of pumpkin seeds on iron, Iranian researchers conducted a small study, providing a daily serving of an iron-rich cereal (providing 7.1 mg of iron per day), along with 30 grams of pumpkin seeds (providing 4.0 mg of iron per day), to eight healthy females of reproductive age (the age of the women is significant, as iron losses from menstrual periods are a major contributor to iron deficiency).[46] After four weeks, the women's iron status improved significantly, but since the researchers did not test the two iron sources separately, it's unknown just how much of the effect was from the cereal and how much was from the pumpkin seeds.

THE BOTTOM LINE

Pumpkin seeds are a quiet nutritional gem that packs a healthy punch: Rich in some often-evasive nutrients, including iron and magnesium, they are also a vegetarian protein source, making them a good choice for the environment. Since they are a seed, pumpkin seeds are usually welcome in nut-free environments, making them a good alternative when almonds, walnuts, pistachios, and peanuts are forbidden. Although only time and research will tell whether eating pumpkin seeds can help prevent certain conditions, including anemia, for now, they stand as a nutritious and easy choice for home or on the road.

SESAME SEEDS

Sesame seeds have a long history in our diets. The problem is they're mostly found on hamburger and hot dog buns. But if you take the sesame seeds away from their less-than-nutritious pals, it turns out those little off-white critters have a lot more to offer than their teeny-tiny size would suggest.

SESAME SEEDS: THE STORY

Sesame (*Sesamun indicum*) is one of the oldest cultivated plants. First grown in Iraq, sesame spread through Asia and Africa and is now found in almost every part of the world with a long growing season. In traditional Asian medicine, sesame is thought to possess anti-aging effects, and it is used medicinally in Taiwan after childbirth. In Ayurvedic medicine, sesame oil is used to treat acne and to improve skin quality. Known for its antibacterial and antifungal properties, sesame oil is thought to be beneficial against skin pathogens, including the athlete's foot fungus and hair lice, and it is used in some parts of Asia and the Middle East to treat diaper rash and to prevent colds and flus by swabbing it inside the nose of schoolchildren. In the United States, Thomas Jefferson is said to have grown sesame, which he referred to by its African name *beni* or *benne*.

Light, golden ivory-brown (white) sesame seeds are grown in Central and South America, including Mexico and Guatemala, while darker (black) sesame seeds are cultivated in Asia, including Thailand and China. In 2009, the biggest producer of sesame seeds in the world was Myanmar (Burma), followed by India and China. Typically, lighter seeds are considered to be of higher quality.

Sesame seeds can be enjoyed on their own or as a tahini, a sesame paste that is commonly used in hummus. The seeds add a nutty flavour (without being a nut) to rice and noodle dishes, stews, and stir-fries. Sesame seeds and oil work well with dark green vegetables and make a great flavour booster for kale, collard greens, and asparagus, to name a few. They are also often found in breads, crackers, melba toast, and muesli, as well as numerous Mediterranean and Middle Eastern dishes, including halva (sesame seed fudge) and Greek pasteli (sesame seed and honey snacks). Unfortunately, sesame seeds can provoke allergies in some individuals. In fact, sesame seeds are one of the 10 priority allergens that are now mandatory on food labels in Canada.[47]

SESAME SEEDS: THE NUTRITION

An ounce of roasted, toasted sesame seeds (28 grams) provides 158 calories, along with 5 grams of protein and 4 grams of fibre. Of their 13 grams of fat, a large proportion (5.8 grams) is derived from omega-6 fatty acids, which is why they don't often show up on heart health lists (as mentioned, it is theorized that our intake of omega-6 fats may be too high relative to our intake of omega-3s, which are derived mostly from fish as well as grass-fed meats, certain types of algae, and in walnuts and flaxseeds). Nonetheless, omega-6s are an essential kind of fat, and if there is trouble from us eating too much, then it's better to reduce our intake from refined and processed foods made with omega-6 fats, such as chips, crackers, and foods fried in the likes of corn, vegetable, sunflower, or safflower oil (all are high in omega-6s), while enjoying all the nutrition benefits of nutrient-dense, unprocessed omega-6-containing foods, such as sesame seeds.

Sesame seeds are rich in energy-producing B vitamins, including vitamin B_1 (providing 15% of your daily value), along with vitamin B_3 (6%), vitamin B_6 (11%), and folate (7%). Their mineral content is where they really shine, however: An ounce of sesame seeds provides 28% of your calcium—that's 277 mg, just shy of the 300 mg in a cup of milk! They are also a terrific way to get your iron, providing 23% of your daily requirements, along with 100 mg of magnesium (25% of your requirements) and 13% of your zinc needs for the day. Now, with that good news comes the reality: Most people won't eat an ounce of sesame seeds, so those numbers won't look nearly as impressive if you're counting on getting your sesame seeds from a hot dog bun.

SESAME SEEDS: THE SCIENCE

If sesame does exert a benefit for the heart or other parts of the body, it is thought that the effect could be the result of compounds known as lignans. Lignans are plant-based compounds that, like pumpkin seeds, have a weak estrogen-like effect that could protect the heart and possibly help improve hormonal status, which could be especially relevant for post-menopausal women. Specifically, sesamin, a type of lignan unique to sesame seeds, is converted to a compound known as enterolactone by bacteria in the intestinal tract. Interestingly, enterolactone is the same compound produced via digestion of flaxseeds, which are also known for their high lignan content.

Although sesame is thought to exert a heart health benefit based on these lignans, what data do we have to prove this? In a study on 33 overweight or obese women given 25 grams of sesame seeds per day for five weeks versus a placebo with an equal number of calories, sesame seeds caused no improvement in lipids (cholesterol, triglycerides) or blood pressure versus placebo.[18] There was also no improvement in any measures of inflammation, such as C-reactive protein, or other inflammatory markers, including interleukin-6 (IL-6) or tumor necrosis factor-alpha.

Fair enough, but perhaps the dose—less than an ounce of sesame seeds—was simply too low to exert a benefit. In a 2006 study, researchers from Taiwan gave 26 healthy post-menopausal women 50 grams of sesame seed powder or a 50-gram rice powder placebo—twice the dose given in the previous study—daily for five weeks.[49] After five weeks, the women on the sesame supplement saw their total cholesterol drop by 5%, LDL ("bad") cholesterol by 10%, and ratio of LDL to HDL ("good") cholesterol improve by 6%, all of which were statistically significant results compared with the start of the study and compared with the placebo. Their LDL cholesterol also demonstrated less damage (oxidation). They also saw a trend to improved hormone status that didn't quite reach statistical significance, but it at least implies that the lignans could do something to minimize symptoms of menopause when consumed in large enough doses. Although this study used large doses (about 2 ounces per day), which may be more than the average person is willing to consume, it at least suggests that sesame seeds have some potential health benefits and could likely work well as part of a diet that includes other nuts and seeds.

LIGNANS VS. LIGNINS

Lignans and lignins are easily confused, and for good reason. *Lignans*, those active compounds found in sesame and flaxseeds, are not actually a form of fibre, and quite frankly, their nutritional significance is not yet fully understood. Although they share the same chemical origins, lignans are much smaller molecules than their homonymous cousins, *lignins*, which are a type of insoluble fibre that makes up part of the walls of plant cells, serving as a form of natural defence. Although lignins are common in many plant foods, lignans are far rarer, usually being found in the bran layer of whole grains or the protective coat of seeds. In fact, the lignan content of most foods is less than 2 mg (0.002 grams) per 100 grams, with two notable exceptions: sesame and flaxseeds. One hundred grams of sesame seeds provide about 373 mg of lignans, and an equal amount of flaxseed provides about 335 mg of lignans.[50] It is this exceptionally high lignan content that is thought to confer some of the unique properties to flaxseeds and sesame seeds and may protect against heart disease and cancer risk.

THE BOTTOM LINE

It's a bit hard to imagine baseball players tossing out their sunflower seeds to munch on teeny-tiny sesame seeds, yet it might make nutritional sense. Fantastically rich in all-important nutrients, including calcium, iron, and magnesium, sesame seeds are far too easily overlooked. Although their effect on human health is only beginning to be understood, sesame seeds deserve more than just to be sprinkled on top of bread.

TOP SUPERFOOD SOURCES OF CALCIUM

FOOD	PORTION	CALCIUM	CALCIUM (% DAILY VALUE)
Sesame seeds, roasted and toasted	1 ounce (28 g)	277 mg	28%
Salba	1 ounce (30 g/2 tbsp)	232 mg	23%
Chia	1 ounce/30 g	177 mg	18%
Amaranth	1 cup, cooked (246 g)	116 mg	12%
Kale	1 cup, raw (67 g)	91 mg	9%

Source: USDA National Nutrient Database (all except Salba, retrieved from www.salbastore.com)

CONCLUSION

So, where do we go from here? In my humble opinion, one of the take-aways from all this is that food is food, and hype is hype. Yes, fruits and vegetables of all kinds are good for you, but if you are being tempted to shell out for an unpronounceable juice at an outrageous price, take my advice: Do not pass GO; head directly to your nearest grocery store, where a carrot awaits you, at a fraction of the cost. And if you heard about the "next big thing" on a TV show, please keep a hold of yourself and go for a walk. Odds are there is more good nutrition in your crisper or freezer right now than you'll get from a mail-order bottle, and you'll save both your wallet and our planet just a little bit if you take the time to prepare it rather than pitch it.

While we devote large amounts of money and text to uncommon and untested juices and potions, I'm one of many who believe we'd do well to remind ourselves of some of the foods that sustained our ancestors for centuries, even millennia. If we get back to raising our animals the way they were meant to be raised, there's a fair case to be made that we might be able to enjoy foods such as beef and cheese again. And while coconut has been a pariah and cocoa seems decadent, the research is finally showing that their long history of use by humans has been founded in more than folklore. Less controversial, but no less nutritious, nuts, seeds, shellfish, berries, and green vegetables have been part of human diets for as long as we've eaten food, and yet they seem easy to forget about when we are presented with a grocery store full of boxes, cartons, and packages. And while drivethroughs and microwaves offer an undeniable convenience, they can also take us farther away from connecting with real, whole food that is more nourishing than anything we can concoct on a lab bench.

So, in the name of all that is whole, I agree with the growing sentiment that we should slow down just a little when it comes to eating. Whether it's learning how to cook green leafy vegetables, experimenting with uncommon whole grains, making your first-ever beet salad, or even just eating at the dinner table with friends or family, there are myriad reasons to revisit our relationship with the meals we make and eat. Odds are, if you read this book, you're making many of these choices already, and that's great. On the other hand, if much of what you read here is new for you, then that's even better: Make today the first day of a new plan for yourself. It's as easy as grabbing a handful of almonds for your next snack. The point of this book is not to argue that there's any one best diet (there are more books making that claim than I could count) but instead to remind people of some of the magic of whole foods—even those without the hype. And that's sensible, decidedly non-headline-generating advice.

ACKNOWLEDGEMENTS

M any thanks go out to Sarah Taylor, for all her help with nutrition-related research, and to Jennifer Forkes, PhD, for helping me understand the environmental consequences of our consumption patterns. I owe a huge debt of gratitude to all the good people at the *National Post*, HarperCollins, and Cleveland Clinic Canada, who had the vision to support a nutrition book that is about evidence, not hyperbole, including Jason Rehel, Ben Errett, Deanna McFadden, Steve Osgoode, Kelly Hope, Brad Wilson, Mike Kessel, Meredith Johnson, Sarah Baker, and Meegan Guest. To all my colleagues at Cleveland Clinic Canada, past and present, especially my good friends in the nutrition department, thanks for bending an ear and lending a hand when I needed it.

Of course, nothing could happen without the phenomenal love and support of my family, who helped in more ways than I could count. I started writing this book when my second son was just over a year old, so to say I needed lots of support is an understatement! So, to my parents, Pam and Gerhard, my husband's parents, Carol and

Charlie, and the two best aunties in the world, Leslie and Jennifer, I could never say thank you enough. So, thank you!

Finally, thank you to my husband, Dave, who is my guardian angel and who carried so much of the load in the year it took to write this book, and to Ben and Ryan, the two funniest, most wonderful humans I've ever known. I love you all.

NOTES

Chapter 1: Overhyped, Overpriced, or Just Plain Bogus

1.   Oz M. "Dr. Oz's Anti-Aging Checklist." From *The Oprah Winfrey Show* Dr. Oz Reveals the Ultimate Checklist for Great Aging (air date February 5, 2008). March 14, 2008. Retrieved from: http://www.oprah.com/health /Dr-Ozs-Ultimate-Anti-Aging-Checklist/3. Accessed May 19, 2013.

2.   Oprah.com. "Dr. Perricone's No. 1 Superfood: Açaí." July 15, 2005. Retrieved from: http://www.oprah.com/health/Acai-Dr-Perricones-No-1-Superfood. Accessed April 18, 2013.

3   Brasileiro A. "'Superfood' Promoted on Oprah's Site Robs Amazon Poor of Staple." Bloomberg.com. May 14, 2009. Retrieved from: http://www .bloomberg.com/apps/news?pid=newsarchive&sid=ai8WCgSJrhmY. Accessed April 18, 2013.

4   Sambazon. "Acai Superfood Juice. Original Acai Juice." Retrieved from: http:// sambazon.com/product/original-acai-juice. Accessed September 6, 2012.

5   Mulabagal V, Keller WJ, Calderón AI. Quantitative analysis of anthocyanins in *Euterpe oleracea* (acai) dietary supplement raw materials and capsules by Q-TOF liquid chromatography/mass spectrometry. *Pharm Biol.* 2012 Aug 20. [Epub ahead of print.]

6   Schauss AG, et al. Phytochemical and nutrient composition of the freeze-dried Amazonian palm berry, *Euterpe oleraceae* Mart. (acai). *J Agric Food Chem.* 2006 Nov 1;54(22):8598–603.

7   United States Department of Agriculture, Agricultural Research Service. "Oxygen Radical Absorbance Capacity (ORAC) of Selected Foods, Release 2 (2010)." Retrieved from: http://www.ars.usda.gov/services/docs.htm?docid =15866. Accessed on April 16, 2013.

8   Seeram NP, et al. Comparison of antioxidant potency of commonly consumed polyphenol-rich beverages in the United States. *J Agric Food Chem.* 2008 Feb 27;56(4):1415–22.

9   Mertens-Talcott SU, et al. Pharmacokinetics of anthocyanins and antioxidant effects after the consumption of anthocyanin-rich acai juice and pulp (*Euterpe oleracea* Mart.) in human healthy volunteers. *J Agric Food Chem.* 2008 Sep 10;56(17):7796–802.

10   Elsayed RK, Glisson JK, Minor DS. Rhabdomyolysis associated with the use of a mislabeled "acai berry" dietary supplement. *Am J Med Sci.* 2011 Dec;342(6):535–8.

11   Heinrich M, Dhanji T, Casselman I. Acai (*Euterpe oleracea* Mart.)—A phytochemical and pharmacological assessment of the species' health claims. *Phytochemistry Letters.* 2011 Mar;4(1):10–21.

12   Thomas J. Letter to Kevin Vokes, MonaVie corporation headquarters. Department of Health and Human Services, Public Health Service, Food and Drug Administration. July 6, 2007. Retrieved from: http://www.fda.gov/down loads/Drugs/GuidanceComplianceRegulatoryInformation/Enforcement ActivitiesbyFDA/CyberLetters/ucm056937.pdf. Accessed September 6, 2012.

13   Dokoupil T. "A Drink's Purple Reign." *Newsweek.* August 1, 2008. Retrieved from: http://www.thedailybeast.com/newsweek/2008/08/01/a-drink-s-purple -reign.html. Accessed April 18, 2013.

14   Oprah.com. "The Truth About Oprah, Dr. Oz, Acai, Resveratrol, Colon Cleanse and More." May 7, 2009. Retrieved from: http://www.oprah.com /health/The-Truth-About-Oprah-Dr-Oz-Acai-Resveratrol-and-Colon -Cleanse. Accessed May 5, 2013.

15   Schardt D. "Web Self-Defense: How to Protect Yourself Against Internet Scams." *Nutrition Action Healthletter.* 2009, April;9–11.

16   Oz M. "Dr. Oz on Men's Health (no. 10 of 19)." From *The Oprah Winfrey Show* 300 Men Ask Dr. Oz (air date October 1, 2007). June 24, 2009. Retrieved from: http://www.oprah.com/health/Dr-Oz-Answers-Mens-Health-Questions/10. Accessed April 18, 2013.

17   Navitas Naturals. "Goji Berries." Retrieved from: http://navitasnaturals.com /product/449/Goji-Berries.html. Accessed April 18, 2013.

18   United States Food and Drug Administration, Department of Health and Human Services, Public Health Service. Letter to Nikki Sandhu, Healthsu perstore.com. August 7, 2006. Retrieved from: http://www.fda.gov/down loads/Drugs/GuidanceComplianceRegulatoryInformation/Enforcement ActivitiesbyFDA/CyberLetters/ucm056356.pdf. Accessed April 18, 2013.

19   Grotto GA, Greenwald GD. In the United States District Court, District of Arizona, David Lucas Burge, Alastair Dick, Lynda Forgette, Pamela Krause, Fred Anthony Reyes, and David Porter Wilson, on behalf of themselves, and a class of persons similarly situated, Plaintiffs, vs. Freeline International, Inc., a Connecticut corporation, Defendant. May 29, 2009. Retrieved from: http://www.gojitrees.com/FreeLifeClassActionLawsuit%5B1%5D.pdf. Accessed April 18, 2013.

20   Health Canada. "Canadian Nutrient File (CNF)—Search by Food." www .hc-sc.gc.ca. Last modified April 26, 2012. Retrieved from: http://webprod3 .hc-sc.gc.ca/cnf-fce/index-eng.jsp. Accessed April 18, 2013.

21   USDA Agricultural Research Service, National Agricultural Library. "National Nutrient Database for Standard Reference. Release 25." Retrieved from: http://ndb.nal.usda.gov. Accessed April 18, 2013.

22   Navitas Naturals. "Goji Berries." Retrieved from: http://navitasnaturals.com /product/449/Goji-Berries.html. Accessed April 18, 2013.

23   Amagase H, Nance DM. A randomized, double-blind, placebo-controlled, clinical study of the general effects of a standardized *Lycium barbarum* (Goji) Juice, GoChi. *J Altern Complement Med.* 2008 May;14(4):403–12.

24   Amagase H, Sun B, Borek C. *Lycium barbarum* (goji) juice improves in vivo antioxidant biomarkers in serum of healthy adults. *Nutr Res.* 2009 Jan;29(1):19–25.

25   Bucheli P, et al. Goji berry effects on macular characteristics and plasma anti-oxidant levels. *Optom Vis Sci.* 2011 Feb;88(2):257–62.

26   Amagase H, Nance DM. *Lycium barbarum* increases caloric expenditure and decreases waist circumference in healthy overweight men and women: pilot study. *J Am Coll Nutr.* 2011 Oct; 30(5):304–9.

27   Health Canada. "Warfarin Interactions with Drugs, Natural Health and Food Products." Last modified October 11, 2005. Retrieved from: http://www .hc-sc.gc.ca/hl-vs/iyh-vsv/med/warfarin-eng.php. Accessed April 18, 2013.

28   Monzon Ballarin S, et al. Anaphylaxis associated with the ingestion of Goji berries (*Lycium barbarum*). *J Investig Allergol Clin Immunol.* 2011;21(7):567–70.

29   Gomez-Bernal S, et al. Systemic photosensitivity due to Goji berries. *Photodermatol Photoimmunol Photomed.* 2011 Oct;27(5):245–7.

30   Wang MY, et al. Morinda citrifolia (noni): a literature review and recent advances in noni research. Acta Pharmacologica Sinica. 2002; 23(12):1127–41.

31   Morinda Bioactives. Tahitian Noni® Original 1-liter. Retrieved from: http:// www.morinda.com/en-us/share/shop/product_detail.html?pid=134. Accessed November 12, 2013.

32   United States Food and Drug Administration, Department of Health and Human Services, Public Health Service. Letter to Sam Chang, Perfect Health, Inc. September 8, 2006. Retrieved from: http://www.fda.gov/downloads /Drugs/GuidanceComplianceRegulatoryInformation/EnforcementActivities byFDA/CyberLetters/ucm056351.pdf. Accessed April 18, 2013.

33   Pawlus AD, Kinghorn AD. Review of the ethnobotany, chemistry, biological activity and safety of the botanical dietary supplement Morinda citrifolia (noni). *J Pharm Pharmacol.* 2007; 59(12):1587–1609.

34   Dussossoy E, et al. Characterization, anti-oxidative and anti-inflammatory effects of Costa Rican noni juice (*Morinda citrifolia* L.). *J Ethnopharmacol.* 2011 Jan 7;133(1):108–15.

35   Ma DL, et al. Evaluation of the ergogenic potential of noni juice. *Phytother Res.* 2007 Nov;21(11):1100–1.

36   Stadlbauer V, et al. Herbal does not at all mean innocuous: the sixth case of hepatotoxicity associated with *Morinda citrifolia* (noni)." *Am J Gastroenterol.* 2008 Sep;103(9):2406–7.

37   Ziobro P. "Coconut Water Brand Vita Coco Sees $100 Million in Sales This Year." *Dow Jones Newswires.* Retrieved from: http://www.advfn.com/nyse /StockNews.asp?stocknews=DPS&article=47732641. Accessed May 4, 2013.

38   Saat M, et al. Rehydration after exercise with fresh young coconut water, carbohydrate-electrolyte beverage and plain water. *J Physiol Anthropol Appl Human Sci.* 2002 Mar;21(2):93–104.

39   Saat M, et al. Rehydration after exercise with fresh young coconut water, carbohydrate-electrolyte beverage and plain water. *J Physiol Anthropol Appl Human Sci.* 2002 Mar;21(2):93–104.

40   Rodriguez NR, et al. Position of the American Dietetic Association, Dietitians of Canada, and the American College of Sports Medicine: Nutrition and Athletic Performance. *J Am Diet Assoc.* 2009;109:509–27.

41   Simpson MR, Howard T. "ACSM Information on Selecting and Effectively Using Hydration for Fitness." American College of Sports Medicine (2011). Retrieved from: http://www.acsm.org/docs/brochures/selecting-and-effec tively-using-hydration-for-fitness.pdf. Accessed May 16, 2013.

42   Rodriguez NR, et al. Position of the American Dietetic Association, Dietitians of Canada, and the American College of Sports Medicine: Nutrition and Athletic Performance. *J Am Diet Assoc.* 2009;109:509–27.

43   Vita Coco. "Vita Coco Congratulates John Isner on Winning the 'Longest Tennis Match in History.'" Businesswire.com (June 24, 2010). Retrieved from: http://www.businesswire.com/news/home/20100624006743/en/Vita

-Coco-Congratulates-John-Isner-Winning-%E2%80%9CLongest. Accessed May 16, 2013.

44   Zelman K. "The Truth About Coconut Water." WebMD.com. Retrieved from: http://www.webmd.com/food-recipes/features/truth-about-coconut-water?page=2. Accessed May 16, 2013.

45   ConsumerLab.com. "Product Review: Coconut Waters Review—Tests of O.N.E., Vita Coco, and Zico." Initial posting August 2, 2011. Retrieved from: https://www.consumerlab.com/reviews/coconut-water-one-vita-coco-zico-review/coconut-water. Accessed May 4, 2013.

46   United States District Court Southern District of New York. Stacy B. Fishbein, Katrina Garcia, Catalina Saldarriaga and Russell Marchewka, on Behalf of Themselves and All Others Similarly Situated, Plaintiffs, v. All Market Inc. d/b/a/ Vita Coco, Defendant. Notice of Class Action and Proposed Settlement. Retrieved from: http://www.vitacocosettlement.com/docs/notice.pdf. Accessed May 4, 2013.

47   Salba, CHIA. "Salba Chia History." Retrieved from: http://www.salbasmart.com/history-of-salba. Accessed April 23, 2013.

48   Salba Founder Mark Gobuty and Salba grower Alfredo Mealla discuss the genesis of Salba. Retrieved from: http://www.youtube.com/watch?v=NwLyxnupNPc. Accessed April 23, 2013.

49   Salba, CHIA. "Products." Retrieved from: http://www.salbasmart.com/salba-seed. Accessed November 12, 2013.

50   Salba, CHIA. "I'm Salba, Smart." Retrieved from: http://www.salbasmart.com. Accessed April 23, 2013.

51   In the United States District Court for the District of Colorado. Salba Corp., N.A., a Canadian corporation, Salba Smart Naturals Products, a Colorado limited liability company, William A. Ralston, and Richard L. Ralston, Plaintiffs, v. X Factor Holdings, LLC, an inactive Florida limited liability company, and Ancient Naturals, LLC, a Florida limited liability company, Defendants. Complaint with Jury Demand. Filed 05/08/12. Retrieved from: http://www.scribd.com/doc/94122448/Salba-Corp-v-X-Factor-Holdings. Accessed April 23, 2013.

52   Ontario Superior Court of Justice. *Mealla v. Salba Corp. N.A.* Court File No. CV-09-8360-00CL. Heard: September 23, 25 and 30, 2009. Judgment: October 1, 2009. Retrieved from: http://fcbarristers.com/Charney/_cases/Mealla%20d1.PDF. Accessed April 23, 2013.

53   Brown L. "Letter to Salba Distributors and Retailers." Re: Response to letters circulated by AgriSalba S.A. or Salba Corp, S.A. August 25, 2009. Retrieved

from: http://chia.typepad.com/files/official_response_agrisalba_fraud_letter
.pdf. Accessed April 23, 2013.

54 Ontario Superior Court of Justice. *Mealla v. Salba Corp. N.A.* Court File
No. CV-09-8360-00CL. Heard: September 23, 25 and 30, 2009. Judgment:
October 1, 2009. Retrieved from: http://fcbarristers.com/Charney/_cases
/Mealla%20d1.PDF. Accessed April 23, 2013.

55 In the United States District Court for the District of Colorado. Salba Corp.,
N.A., a Canadian corporation, Salba Smart Naturals Products, a Colorado
limited liability company, William A. Ralston, and Richard L. Ralston,
Plaintiffs, v. X Factor Holdings, LLC, an inactive Florida limited liability
company, and Ancient Naturals, LLC, a Florida limited liability company,
Defendants. Complaint with Jury Demand. Filed 05/08/12. Retrieved from:
http://www.scribd.com/doc/94122448/Salba-Corp-v-X-Factor-Holdings.
Accessed April 23, 2013.

56 In the United States District Court for the District of Colorado. Salba Corp.,
N.A., a Canadian corporation, Salba Smart Naturals Products, a Colorado
limited liability company, William A. Ralston, and Richard L. Ralston, Plaintiffs, v. X Factor Holdings, LLC, an inactive Florida limited liability company,
and Ancient Naturals, LLC, a Florida limited liability company, Defendants.
Minute Order. Filed 03/18/2013. Retrieved from: http://archive.recapthelaw
.org/cod/133340. Accessed April 23, 2013.

57 Salba, CHIA. "Salba Chia Nutrition." Retrieved from: http://www.sal
basmart.com/salba-nutrition. Accessed April 24, 2013.

58 Vuksan V, et al. Reduction in postprandial glucose excursion and prolongation
of satiety: possible explanation of the long-term effects of whole grain Salba
(*Salvia Hispanica* L.). *Eur J Clin Nutr.* 2010 Apr;64(4):436–8.

59 Vuksan V, et al. Supplementation of conventional therapy with the novel grain
Salba (*Salvia Hispanica* L.) improves major and emerging cardiovascular risk
factors in type 2 diabetes: results of a randomized controlled trial. *Diabetes
Care.* 2007 Nov;30(11):2804–10.

60 Forbes.com. "The world's billionaires: Stewart and Lynda Resnick." March
2013. Retrieved from: http://www.forbes.com/profile/stewart-and-lyn
da-resnick. Accessed April 14, 2013.

61 Melnick M. "FTC and FDA to POM: you're not so wonderful." *Time.* September. 27, 2010. Retrieved from: http://healthland.time.com/2010/09/27
/ftc-and-fda-to-pom-youre-not-quite-so-wonderful. Accessed April 14, 2013.

62 Wernau J. "FTC: POM Wonderful health claims are bogus." *Chicago Tri-
bune.* September 27, 2010. Retrieved from: http://www.chicagotribune.com
/health/ct-pom-juice-story,0,7571209.story. Accessed April 14, 2013.

63 Federal Trade Commission. "FTC Complaint Charges Deceptive Advertising by POM Wonderful." September 27, 2010. Retrieved from: http://www.ftc .gov/opa/2010/09/pom.shtm. Accessed April 14, 2013.

64 United States of America, Federal Trade Commission, Office of Administrative Law Judges, Docket No. 9344. In the matter of Pom Wonderful LLC and Roll Global LLC, as successor in interest to Roll International Corporation, companies, and Stewart A. Resnick, Lynda Rae Resnick, and Matthew Tupper, individually and as officers of the companies, Respondents. Initial Decision. May 17, 2012. Retrieved from: http://www.ftc.gov/os/adjpro/d9344/120521pom decision.pdf. Accessed April 14, 2013.

65 United States of America Before the Federal Trade Commission. In the Matter of Pom Wonderful LLC and Roll Global LLC, as successor in interest to Roll International Corporation, companies, and Stewart A. Resnick, Lynda Rae Resnick, and Matthew Tupper, individually and as officers of the companies, Respondents. Opinion of the Commission. Filed 01/10/13. Retrieved from: http://www.ftc.gov/os/adjpro/d9344/130116pomopinion .pdf. Accessed April 18, 2013.

66 Federal Trade Commission. FTC Commissioners Uphold Trial Judge Decision that POM Wonderful, LLC; Stewart and Lynda Resnick; Others Deceptively Advertised Pomegranate Products by Making Unsupported Health Claims. Released 01/16/2013. Retrieved from: http://www.ftc.gov /opa/2013/01/pom.shtm. Accessed April 18, 2013.

67 United States Court of Appeals, District of Columbia Circuit. Pom Wonderful LLC and Roll Global LLC, as successor in interest to Roll International Corporation, companies, and Stewart A. Resnick, Lynda Rae Resnick, and Matthew Tupper, individually and as officers of the companies, Petitioners. V. Federal Trade Commission, Respondent. Petition for Review. Filed 03/08/2013. Retrieved from: http://www.hpm.com/pdf/blog/POM%20-%20Petition%20 for%20Review%20DC%20Cir.pdf. Accessed April 18, 2013.

68 Aviram M, et al. Pomegranate juice consumption reduces oxidative stress, atherogenic modifications to LDL, and platelet aggregation: studies in humans and in atherosclerotic apolipoprotein-deficient mice. *Am J Clin Nutr.* 2000 May;71(5):1062–76.

69 Aviram M, Dornfield L. Pomegranate juice consumption inhibits serum angiotensin converting enzyme activity and reduces systolic blood pressure. *Atherosclerosis.* 2001 Sep;158(1):195–8.

70 González-Ortiz M, et al. Effect of pomegranate juice on insulin secretion and sensitivity in patients with obesity. *Ann Nutr Metab.* 2011;58(3):220–3.

71 Barrett A, et al. Inhibition of α-amlyase and glucoamylase by tannins extracted

from cocoa, pomegranates, cranberries, and grapes. *J Agric Food Chem.* 2013 Feb 20;61(7):1477–86.

72   Trombold JR, et al. The effect of pomegranate juice supplementation on strength and soreness after eccentric exercise. *J Strength Cond Res.* 2011 Jul;25(7):1782–8.

73   Trombold JR, et al. Ellagitannin consumption improves strength recovery 2–3 d after eccentric exercise. *Med Sci Sports Exerc.* 2010 Mar;42(3):493–9.

Chapter 2: Quinoa, I Thought I Knew Ya

1   Schlick G, Bubenheim DL. Quinoa: An Emerging "New" Crop with Potential for CELSS. NASA Technical Paper 3422. November 1993.

2   Green P, Hemming C. *Quinoa 365: The Everyday Superfood.* (Vancouver) Whitecap Books Ltd., 2010.

3   Gonzalez JA, et al. Interrelationships among seed yield, total protein and amino acid composition of ten quinoa (*Chenopodium quinoa*) cultivars from two different agroecological regions. *J Sci Food Agric.* 2012 Apr;92(6):1222–9.

4   Zevallos VF, et al. Variable activation of immune response by quinoa (*Chenopodium quinoa* Willd.) prolamins in celiac disease. *Am J Clin Nutr.* 2012 Aug;96(2):337–44.

5   United Nations Food and Agriculture Organization. "Quinoa 2013 International Year: Frequently Asked Questions." Retrieved from: http://www.fao .org/quinoa-2013/faqs/en. Accessed November 12, 2013.

6   Candela G. "Quinoa, Bolivia's golden grain." InfoSurHoy. December 20, 2012. Retrieved from: http://infosurhoy.com/en_GB/articles/saii/features/econ omy/2012/12/20/feature-02. Accessed January 8, 2013.

7   Friedman-Rudovsky J. "Quinoa: The dark side of an Andean superfood." *Time.* April 3, 2012. Retrieved from: http://content.time.com/time/world /article/0,8599,2110890-1,00.html. Accessed January 8, 2013.

8   Romero S, Shahriari S. "Quinoa's global success creates quandary at home." *New York Times.* March 19, 2011. Retrieved from: http://www.nytimes .com/2011/03/20/world/americas/20bolivia.html?_r=4&. Accessed January 8, 2013.

9   Bland A. "Quinoa craze inspires North America to start growing its own." National Public Radio, The Salt. November 29, 2012. Retrieved from: http:// www.npr.org/blogs/thesalt/2012/11/29/166155875/quinoa-craze-in spires-north-america-to-start-growing-its-own?utm_source=NPR&utm_ medium=facebook&utm_campaign=20121129#1. Accessed January 8, 2013.

10   Joseph Enterprises. "Chia Products." Retrieved from: http://www.chiapet .com/index.php/chia-products. Accessed November 18, 2012.

11   Jin F, et al. Supplementation of milled chia seeds increases plasma ALA and EPA in postmenopausal women. *Plant Foods Hum Nutr.* 2012 Jun;67(2):105–10.

12   Antruejo A, et al. Omega-3 enriched egg production: the effect of α-linoleic ω-3fatty acid sources on laying hen performance and yolk lipid content and fatty acid composition. *British Poultry Science.* 2011;52(6):750–60.

13   Mohd Ali N, et al. The promising future of chia, *Salvia hispanica* L. *J Biomed Biotechnol.* [Epub November 21, 2012].

14   Ayerza R, Coates W. Effect of dietary α-linolenic fatty acid derived from chia when fed as ground seed, whole seed and oil on lipid content and fatty acid composition of rat plasma. *Ann Nutr Metab.* 2007;51(1):27–34.

15   Guevara-Cruz M, et al. A dietary pattern including nopal, chia seed, soy protein, and oat reduces serum triglycerides and improves glucose tolerance in patients with metabolic syndrome. *J Nutr.* 2012 Jan;142(1):64–9.

16   Nieman DC, et al. Chia seed does not promote weight loss or alter disease risk factors in overweight adults. *Nutr Res.* 2009 Jun;29(6):414–8.

17   Niemen DC, et al. Chia seed supplementation and disease risk factors in overweight women: a metabolomics investigation. *J Altern Complement Med.* 2012 Jul;18(7):700–8.

18   Illian TG, et al. Omega 3 chia seed loading as a means of carbohydrate loading. *J Strength Cond Res.* 2011 Jan;25(1):61–5.

19   Mount S. "Answers from the FAQ, Page 8 Q145." "What kind of paper was the Constitution written on?" USConstitution.net. Last modified January 24, 2010. Retrieved from: http://www.usconstitution.net/constfaq_a8.html. Accessed April 24, 2013.

20   U.S. Department of Agriculture. "Hemp for Victory." Uploaded August 15, 2010. Retrieved from: http://www.youtube.com/watch?v=W0xHCk Onn-A. Accessed April 24, 2013.

21   Editorial. "Give this plant its due: legalize hemp." *Los Angeles Times.* February 25, 2013. Retrieved from: http://articles.latimes.com/2013/feb/25/opinion /la-ed-hemp-legalize-cultivation-congress-20130225. Accessed April 24, 2013.

22   Manitoba Harvest Hemp Foods. "Hemp History Timeline." Manitobahar vest.com. Retrieved from: http://manitobaharvest.com/about_hemp/3775 /Hemp-History.html. Accessed April 24, 2013.

23   Agriculture and Agri-Food Canada. "Industrial Hemp. Profile: Canada's Industrial Hemp Industry." www.agr.gc.ca. Last updated March 22, 2007. Retrieved from: http://www4.agr.gc.ca/AAFC-AAC/display-afficher .do?id=1174595656066&lang=eng. Accessed April 24, 2013.

24   Kupetsky-Rincon EA, Uitto J. Magnesium: novel applications in cardiovascular disease—a review of the literature. *Ann Nutr Metab.* 2012;61(2):102–10.

25   Health Canada. "Do Canadian Adults Meet Their Nutrient Requirements Through Food Intake Alone?" Retrieved from: http://www.hc-sc.gc.ca/fn-an /surveill/nutrition/commun/art-nutr-adult-eng.php. Accessed April 3, 2013.

26   Simopoulos AP. The importance of the omega-6/omega-3 fatty acid ratio in cardiovascular disease and other chronic diseases. *Exp Biol Med (Maywood)*. 2008 Jun;233(6):674–88.

27   Kuipers RS, et al. Estimated macronutrient and fatty acid intakes from an East African Paleolithic diet. *Br J Nutr*. 2010 Dec;104(11):1666–87.

28   Simopoulos AP. The importance of the omega-6/omega-3 fatty acid ratio in cardiovascular disease and other chronic diseases. *Exp Biol Med (Maywood)*. 2008 Jun;233(6):674–88.

29   Harris WS, et al. Omega-6 fatty acids and risk for cardiovascular disease: a science advisory from the American Heart Association Subcommittee of the Council on Nutrition, Physical Activity, and Metabolism; Council on Cardio-vascular Nursing; and Council on Epidemiology and Prevention. *Circulation*. 2009 Feb 17;119(6):902–7.

30   Lee SP, et al. Effect of altering dietary n-6:n-3 PUFA ratio on cardiovascular disease risk measures in patients treated with statins: a pilot study. *Br J Nutr*. 2012 Oct;108(7):1280–5.

31   Chen T, et al. The isolation and identification of two compounds with pre-dominant radical scavenging activity in hempseed (seed of *Cannabis sativa* L.). *Food Chem*. 2012 Sep 15;134(2):1030–7.

32   Lee MJ, et al. The effects of hempseed meal intake and linoleic acid on *Drosophila* models of neurodegenerative diseases and hypercholesterolemia. *Mol Cells*. 2011 Apr;31(4):337–42.

33   Al-Khalifa A, et al. Effect of dietary hempseed intake on cardiac ischemia-reperfusion injury. *Am J Physiol Regul Integr Comp Physiol*. 2007 Mar;292(3):1198–203.

34   Prociuk MA, et al. Cholesterol-induced stimulation of platelet aggregation is prevented by a hempseed-enriched diet. *Can J Physiol Pharmacol*. 2008 Apr;86(4):153–9.

35   Saberivand A, et al. The effects of *Cannabis sativa* L. seed (hempseed) in the ovarectomized rat model of menopause. *Methods Find Exp Clin Pharmacol*. 2010 Sep;32(7):467–73.

36   Callaway J, et al. Efficacy of dietary hempseed oil in patients with atopic dermatitis. *J Dermatolog Treat*. 2005 Apr;16(2):87–94.

37   Agriculture and Agri-Food Canada. "Industrial Hemp. Profile: Canada's Industrial Hemp Industry." www.agr.gc.ca. Last updated March 22, 2007.

Retrieved from: http://www4.agr.gc.ca/AAFC-AAC/display-afficher .do?id=1174595656066&lang=eng. Accessed April 24, 2013.

38   Encyclopedia Britannica. "Coconut palm." Britannica.com. Retrieved from: http://www.britannica.com/EBchecked/topic/123794/coconut-palm#ref151445 (membership required). Accessed May 15, 2013.

39   Prior IA. Cholesterol, coconuts, and diet on Polynesian atolls: a natural experiment: the Pukapuka and Tokelau Island studies. *Am J Clin Nutr.* 1981;34(8):1552–61.

40   Mendis S, Kumarasunderam R. The effect of daily consumption of coconut fat and soya-bean fat on plasma lipids and lipoproteins of young normolipidemic men. *Br J Nutr.* 1990 May;63(3):547–52.

41   Mendis S, Samarajeewa U, Thattil RO. Coconut fat and serum lipoproteins: effects of partial replacement with unsaturated fats. *Br J Nutr.* 2001 May;85(5):583–9.

42   Kumar PD, et al. The role of coconut and coconut oil in coronary heart disease in Kerala, south India. *Trop Doct.* 1997 Oct;27(4):215–7.

43   Lipoeto NI, et al. Dietary intake and the risk of coronary heart disease among the coconut-consuming Minangkabau in West Sumatra, Indonesia. *Asia Pac J Clin Nutr.* 2004;13(4):377–84.

44   Lipoeto NI, et al. Dietary intake and the risk of coronary heart disease among the coconut-consuming Minangkabau in West Sumatra, Indonesia. *Asia Pac J Clin Nutr.* 2004;13(4):377–84.

45   Assunção, ML, et al. Effects of dietary coconut oil on the biochemical and anthropometric profiles of women presenting abdominal obesity. *Lipids.* 2009 Jul;44(7):593–601.

46   Feranil AB, et al. Coconut oil is associated with a beneficial lipid profile in pre-menopausal women in the Philippines. *Asia Pac J Clin Nutr.* 2011;20(2):190–5.

47   Müller H, et al. The serum LDL/HDL cholesterol ratio is influenced more favorably by exchanging saturated with unsaturated fat than by reducing saturated fat in the diet of women. *J Nutr.* 2003 Jan;133(1):78-83.

48   St-Onge MP, Bosarge A. Weight-loss diet that includes consumption of medium-chain triacylglycerol oil leads to a greater rate of weight and fat mass loss than does olive oil. *Am J Clin Nutr.* 2008 Mar;87(3):621–6.

49   St-Onge MP, et al. Medium chain triglyceride oil consumption as part of a weight loss diet does not lead to an adverse metabolic profile when compared to olive oil. *J Am Coll Nutr.* 2008 Oct;27(5):547–52.

50   Liau KM, et al. An open-label pilot study to assess the efficacy and safety

of virgin coconut oil in reducing visceral adiposity. *ISRN Pharmacol.* 2011;2011:94949686.

51 De Laurentiis G. "Grilled Salmon with Citrus Salsa Verde." Foodnetwork .com. Retrieved from: http://www.foodnetwork.com/recipes/giada-de-lau rentiis/grilled-salmon-with-citrus-salsa-verde-recipe/index.html. Accessed May 14, 2013.

52 The University of Sydney. "Agave." Glycemicindex.com. Last updated June 21, 2012. Retrieved from: http://www.glycemicindex.com/foodSearch.php. Accessed May 14, 2013.

53 Willems JL, Low NH. Major carbohydrate, polyol, and oligosaccharide pro-files of agave syrup. Application of this data to authenticity analysis. *J Agric Food Chem.* 2012 Sep 5;60(35):8745–54.

54 Weil A. "What's Wrong with Agave Nectar?" Drweil.com. September 4, 2012. Retrieved from: http://www.drweil.com/drw/u/QAA401166/Whats -Wrong-with-Agave-Nectar.html. Accessed May 14, 2013.

55 Basciano H, Federico L, Khosrow A. Fructose, insulin resistance, and meta-bolic dyslipidemia. *Nutr Metab.* 2005;2:5.

56 Sievenpiper JL, et al. Heterogeneous effects of fructose on blood lipids in indi-viduals with type 2 diabetes: systematic review and meta-analysis of experi-mental trials in humans. *Diabetes Care.* 2009 Oct;32(10):1930–7.

57 Sievenpiper JL, et al. Effect of fructose on body weight in controlled feed-ing trials: a systematic review and meta-analysis. *Ann Intern Med.* 2012 Feb 21;156(4):291–304.

58 Cozma AI, et al. Effect of fructose on glycemic control in diabetes: a system-atic review and meta-analysis of controlled feeding trials. *Diabetes Care.* 2012 Jul;35(7):1611–20.

59 Figlewicz DP, et al. Effect of moderate intake of sweeteners on metabolic health in the rat. *Physiol Behav.* 2009 Dec 7;98(5):618–24.

60 Urías-Silvas JE, et al. Physiological effects of dietary fructans extracted from *Agave tequilana* Gto. and *Dasylirion* spp. *Br J Nutr.* 2008 Feb;99(2):254–61.

61 Mellado-Mojica F, López MG. Fructan metabolism in *A. tequilana* Weber Blue variety along its developmental cycle in the field. *J Agric Food Chem.* 2012 Nov 28;60(47):11704–13.

62 Johannes L. "Agave syrup may not be so simple." *Wall Street Journal.* October 27, 2009. Retrieved from: http://online.wsj.com/article/SB1000142405274 8704335904574497622806733800.html. Accessed May 22, 2013.

63 Núñez HM, Rodríguez LF, Khanna M. Agave for tequila and biofuels: an economic assessment and potential opportunities. *GCB Bioenergy.* 2011 Feb;3(1):43–57.

64   Garcia-Moya E, Romero-Manzanares A, Nobel PS. Highlights for agave productivity. *GCB Bioenergy.* 2011 Feb;3(1):4–14.

65   Architectural and Historical Research, LLC. "Historic Overview: The American Butter Company Building." Ahr-kc.com. 2010. Retrieved from: http://ahr-kc.com/reports/american_butter_company. Accessed February 27, 2013.

66   Architectural and Historical Research, LLC. "Historic Overview: The American Butter Company Building." Ahr-kc.com. 2010. Retrieved from: http://ahr-kc.com/reports/american_butter_company. Accessed February 27, 2013.

67   PINES The Wheat Grass People. "The History of Wheatgrass." Wheatgrass.com. Retrieved from: http://www.wheatgrass.com/t-the-history-of-wheat grass.aspx. Accessed February 27, 2013.

68   PINES The Wheat Grass People. "Nutritional Analysis of Fresh Wheatgrass Juice." Wheatgrass.com. Retrieved from: http://www.wheatgrass.com/t -nutritional-analysis-fresh-wheatgrass-juice.aspx. Accessed April 24, 2013.

69   PINES The Wheat Grass People. "Nutritional Analysis of Fresh Wheatgrass Juice." Wheatgrass.com. Retrieved from: http://www.wheatgrass.com/t -nutritional-analysis-fresh-wheatgrass-juice.aspx. Accessed April 24, 2013.

70   Kothari S, et al. Hypolipidemic effect of fresh *Triticum aestivum* (wheat) grass juice in hypercholesterolemic rats. *Acta Pol Pharm.* 2011 Mar-Apr;68(2):291–4.

71   Elvehjem CA, et al. A new essential dietary factor. *J Biol Chem.* 1936;115:707.

72   Kohler GO, Elvehjem CA, Hart EB. Further studies on the growth promoting factor associated with summer milk. *J Nutr.* 1937;14:131–44.

73   *JAMA.* 1939;113(5):446.

74   Ben-Arye E, et al. Wheat grass juice in the treatment of active distal ulcerative colitis: a randomized double-blind placebo-controlled trial. *Scand J Gastroenterol.* 2002 Apr;37(4):444–9.

75   Marwaha RK, et al. Wheat grass juice reduces transfusion requirements in patients with thalassemia major: a pilot study. *Indian Pediatr.* 2004 Jul;41(7):716–20.

76   Choudhary DR, et al. Effect of wheat grass therapy on transfusion requirement in beta-thalassemia major. *Indian J Pediatr.* 2009 Apr;76(4):375–6.

77   Kothari S, et al. Hypolipidemic effect of fresh *Triticum aestivum* (wheat) grass juice in hypercholesterolemic rats. *Acta Pol Pharm.* 2011 Mar-Apr;68(2):291–4.

78   Kothari S, et al. Effect of fresh *Triticum aestivum* grass juice on lipid profile of normal rats. *Indian J Pharmacol.* 2008 Oct;40(5):235–6.

79   Sethi J, et al. Antioxidant effect of *Triticum aestivium* (wheat grass) in high-fat diet-induced oxidative stress in rabbits. *Methods Fin Exp Clin Pharmacol.* 2010 May;32(4):233–5.

80   Bar-Sela G, et al. Wheat grass juice may improve hematological toxicity

related to chemotherapy in breast cancer patients: a pilot study. *Nutr Cancer.* 2007;58(1):43–8.

Chapter 3: Smear Campaign

1   Noakes M, et al. Effect of an energy-restricted, high-protein, low-fat diet relative to a conventional high-carbohydrate, low-fat diet on weight loss, body composition, nutritional status, and markers of cardiovascular health in obese women. *Am J Clin Nutr.* 2005 Jun;81(6):1298–306.

2   Clifton PM, Bastiaans K, Keogh JB. High protein diets decrease total and abdominal fat and improve CVD risk profile in overweight and obese men and women with elevated triacylglycerol. *Nutr Metab Cardiovasc Dis.* 2009 Oct;19(8):548–54.

3   Wolfe BM, Piché LA. Replacement of carbohydrate by protein in a conventional-fat diet reduces cholesterol and triglyceride concentrations in healthy normolipidemic subjects. *Clin Invest Med.* 1999 Aug;22(4):140–8.

4   Krauss RM, et al. Separate effects of reduced carbohydrate intake and weight loss on atherogenic dyslipidemia. *Am J Clin Nutr.* 2006 May;83(5):1025–31.

5   Furtado JD, et al. Effect of protein, unsaturated fat, and carbohydrate intakes on plasma apolipoprotein B and VLDL and LDL containing apolipoprotein C-III: results from the OmniHeart Trial. *Am J Clin Nutr.* 2008 June;87(6):1623–30.

6   Astrup A, et al. The role of reducing intakes of saturated fat in the prevention of cardiovascular disease: where does the evidence stand in 2010? *Am J Clin Nutr.* 2011 Apr;93(4):684–8.

7   Lawrence GD. Dietary fats and health: dietary recommendations in the context of scientific evidence. *Adv Nutr.* 2013 May 1;4(3);294–302.

8   Siri-Tarino PH, et al. Saturated fatty acids and risk of coronary heart disease: modulation by replacement nutrients. *Curr Atheroscler Rep.* 2010 Nov;12(6):384–90.

9   Wolfe BM, Giovannetti PM. Short-term effects of substituting protein for carbohydrates in the diets of moderately hypercholesterolemic human subjects. *Metabolism.* 1991 Apr;40(4):338–43.

10 Siri-Tarino PH, et al. Saturated fatty acids and risk of coronary heart disease: modulation by replacement nutrients. *Curr Atheroscler Rep.* 2010 Nov;12(6):384–90.

11 Micha R, Wallace SK, Mozaffarian D. Red and processed meat consumption and risk of incident coronary heart disease, stroke, and diabetes: a systematic review and meta-analysis. *Circulation.* 2010 June 1;121(21):2271–83.

12 Fretts AM, et al. Associations of processed meat and unprocessed red meat intake with incident diabetes: the Strong Heart Family Study. *Am J Clin Nutr.* 2012 Mar;95(3):752–8.

13 Pollan M. *The Omnivore's Dilemma: A Natural History of Four Meals*. New York: Penguin Press, 2006.

14 Daley CA, et al. A review of fatty acid profiles and antioxidant content in grass-fed and grain-fed beef. *Nutr J*. 2010 Mar 10;9:10.

15 World Cancer Research Fund/American Institute for Cancer Research. *Food, Nutrition, Physical Activity, and the Prevention of Cancer: A Global Perspective*. Washington, DC: AICR, 2007.

16 Symons TB, et al. A moderate serving of high-quality protein maximally stimulates skeletal muscle protein synthesis in young and elderly subjects. *J Am Diet Assoc*. 2009 Sep;109(9):1582–6.

17 Paddon-Jones D, Rasmussen BB. Dietary recommendations and the prevention of sarcopenia. *Curr Opin Clin Nutr Metab Care*. 2009 Jan;12(1):86–90.

18 Volpi E, et al. Is the optimal level of protein intake for older adults greater than the recommended dietary allowance? *J Gerontol A Biol Sci Med Sci*. 2012 Nov 26. [Epub ahead of print.]

19 Benatar JR, Sidhu K Stewart RA. Effects of high and low fat dairy food on cardio-metabolic risk factors: a meta-analysis of randomized studies. *PLoS One*. 2013 Oct 11;8(10):e76480.

20 Soedamah-Muthu SS, et al. Milk and dairy consumption and incidence of cardiovascular diseases and all-cause mortality: dose-response meta-analysis of prospective cohort studies. *Am J Clin Nutr*. 2011 Jan;93(1):158–71.

21 Louie JC, et al. Higher regular fat dairy consumption is associated with lower incidence of metabolic syndrome but not type 2 diabetes. *Nutr Metab Cardiovasc Dis*. 2013 Sep;23(9):816–21.

22 Nestel PJ, et al. Effects of low-fat or full-fat fermented and non-fermented dairy foods on selected cardiovascular biomarkers in overweight adults. *Br J Nutr*. 2013 Jun 12;1–8.

23 Sonestedt E, et al. Dairy products and its association with incidence of cardiovascular disease: the Malmö diet and cancer cohort. *Eur J Epidemiol*. 2011 Aug;26(8):609–18.

24 Patterson E, et al. Association between dairy food consumption and risk of myocardial infarction in women differs by type of dairy food. *J Nutr*. 2013 Jan;143(1):74–9.

25 Geleijnse JM, et al. Dietary intake of menaquinone is associated with a reduced risk of coronary heart disease: the Rotterdam study. *J Nutr*. 2004; 134:3100–5.

26 Gast GCM, et al. A high menaquinone intake reduces the incidence of coronary heart disease. *Nutr Metab Cardiovasc Dis*. 2009 Sep;19(7):504–10.

27 Cockayne S, et al. Vitamin K and the prevention of fractures: systematic review and meta-analysis of randomized controlled trials. *Arch Intern Med*. 2006 Jun 26;166(12):1256–61.

28 Samykutty A, et al. Vitamin K$_2$, a naturally occurring menaquinone, exerts therapeutic effects on both hormone-dependent and hormone-independent prostate cancer cells. *Evid Based Complement Alternat Med.* 2013 Aug 24;2013:287358. [Epub]

29 Larsson SC, Bergkvist L, Wolk A. High-fat dairy food and conjugated linoleic acid intakes in relation to colorectal cancer incidence in the Swedish Mammography Cohort. *Am J Clin Nutr.* 2005 Oct;82(4):894–900.

30 Shearer MJ, Bach A, Kohlmeier M. Chemistry, nutritional sources, tissue distribution and metabolism of vitamin K with special reference to bone health. *J Nutr.* 1996 Apr;126 Suppl 4: S1181–6.

31 Kamao, M, et al. Vitamin K content of foods and dietary vitamin K intake in Japanese young women. *J Nutr Sci Vitaminol.* 2007 Dec;53(6):464-70.

32 Kamao et al, 2007.

33 Dillinger TL, et al. Food of the gods: cure for humanity? A cultural history of the medicinal and ritual use of chocolate. *J Nutr.* 2000 Aug;130(8):S2057–72.

34 Dillinger TL, et al. Food of the gods: cure for humanity? A cultural history of the medicinal and ritual use of chocolate. *J Nutr.* 2000 Aug;130(8):S2057–72.

35 Hollenberg NK, et al. Aging, acculturation, salt intake, and hypertension in the Kuna of Panama. *Hypertension.* 1997;29:197–76.

36 Corti R, et al. Cocoa and cardiovascular health. *Circulation.* 2009;119:1433–41.

37 Ried K, et al. Effect of cocoa on blood pressure. *Cochrane Database Syst Rev.* 2012 Aug 15;8:CD008893.

38 Buijsse B, et al. Cocoa intake, blood pressure, and cardiovascular mortality: the Zutphen Elderly Study. *Arch Intern Med.* 2006;166:411–17.

39 Hooper L, et al. Effects of chocolate, cocoa, and flavan-3-ols on cardiovascular health: a systematic review and meta-analysis of randomized trials. *Am J Clin Nutr.* 2012 Mar;95(3):740–51.

40 Tokede OA, Gaziano JM, Djoussé L. Effects of cocoa products/dark chocolate on serum lipids: a meta-analysis. *Eur J Clin Nutr.* 2011 Aug;65(8):879–86.

41 Faridi Z, et al. Acute dark chocolate and cocoa ingestion and endothelial function: a randomized controlled crossover trial. *Am J Clin Nutr.* 2008 Jul;88(1):58–63.

42 Landberg R, Naidoo N, van Dam RM. Diet and endothelial function: from individual components to dietary patterns. *Curr Opin Lipidol.* 2012 Apr;23(2):147–55.

43 Dillinger TL, et al. Food of the gods: cure for humanity? A cultural history of the medicinal and ritual use of chocolate. *J Nutr.* 2000 Aug;130(8):S2057–72.

44 Schardt D. How bittersweet it is. *Nutrition Action Healthletter.* December 2013:8–10.

45   Spence JD, Jenkins DJ, Davignon J. Dietary cholesterol and egg yolks: not for patients at risk of vascular disease. *Can J Cardiol.* 2010 Nov;26(9):e336–9.

46   Sommerburg O, et al. Fruits and vegetables that are sources for lutein and zeaxanthin: the macular pigment in human eyes. *Br J Ophthalmol.* 1998;82:907–10.

47   Burnbrae Farms. "Naturegg Omega Pro." Burnbraefarms.com. Retrieved from: http://www.burnbraefarms.com/consumer/our_products/shell_naturegg_omega_pro.htm#. Accessed February 13, 2013.

48   Conis, E. "Enriched eggs, milk may not be best source for omega-3." *Los Angeles Times.* December 13, 2010. Retrived from: http://articles.latimes.com/print/2010/dec/13/health/la-he-nutrition-lab-omega-20101213. Accessed February 13, 2013.

49   Hu FB, et al. A prospective study of egg consumption and risk of cardiovascular disease in men and women. *JAMA.* 1999 Apr 21;281(15):1387–94.

50   Centers for Disease Control and Prevention (CDC). Surveillance for foodborne disease outbreaks—United States, 2009–2010. *MMWR Morb Mortal Wkly Rep.* 2013 Jan 25;62(3):41–7.

51   Health Canada. "Tips for Using Eggs Safely." hc-sc.gc.ca. Last modified April 18, 2011. Retrieved from: http://www.hc-sc.gc.ca/fn-an/securit/kitchen-cuisine/eggs-oeufs-eng.php. Accessed April 25, 2013.

52   Qureshi AI, et al. Regular egg consumption does not increase the risk of stroke and cardiovascular diseases. *Med Sci Monit.* 2007 Jan;13(1):CR1–8.

53   Houston DK, et al. Dietary fat and cholesterol and risk of cardiovascular disease in older adults: the Health ABC Study. *Nutr Metab Cardiovasc Dis.* 2011 June;21(6):430–7.

54   Pearce KL, Clifton PM, Noakes M. Egg consumption as part of an energy-restricted high-protein diet improves blood lipid and blood glucose profiles in individuals with type 2 diabetes. *Br J Nutr.* 2011 Feb;105(4):584–92.

55   Hu FB, Manson JE, Willett WC. Types of dietary fat and risk of coronary heart disease: a critical overview. *J Am Coll Nutr.* 2001 Feb;20(1):5–19.

56   Houston DK, et al. Dietary fat and cholesterol and risk of cardiovascular disease in older adults: the Health ABC Study. *Nutr Metab Cardiovasc Dis.* 2011 June;21(6):430–7.

57   Howell WH, et al. Plasma lipid and lipoprotein responses to dietary fat and cholesterol: a meta-analysis. *Am J Clin Nutr.* 1997 June;65(6):1747–64.

58   Encyclopedia Britannica. "George Washington Carver." Britannica.com. Retrieved from: http://www.britannica.com/EBchecked/topic/97606/George-Washington-Carver (membership required). Accessed May 10, 2013.

59   Reis CE, et al. Acute and second-meal effects of peanuts on glycaemic response and appetite in obese women with high type 2 diabetes risk: a randomized cross-over clinical trial. *Br J Nutr.* 2012 Nov 5:1–9.

60   McKiernan F, et al. Effects of peanut processing on body weight and fasting plasma lipids. *Br J Nutr.* 2010 Aug;104(3):418–26.

61   Kris-Etherton PM, et al. High-monounsaturated fatty acid diets lower both plasma cholesterol and triacylglycerol concentrations. *Am J Clin Nutr.* 1999 Dec;70(6):1009–15.

62   Varshney P, et al. A randomized controlled study of peanut oral immunotherapy (OIT): clinical desensitization and modulation of the allergic response. *J Allergy Clin Immunol.* 2011 Mar;127(3):654–60.

63   Nurmatov U, et al. Allergen-specific oral immunotherapy for peanut allergy. *Cochrane Database Syst Rev.* 2012 Sep 12;9:CD009014.

64   Pruser KN, Flynn NE. Acrylamide in health and disease. *Front Biosci (Schol Ed).* 2011 Jan 1;3:41–51.

65   Randi G, et al. Dietary patterns and the risk of colorectal cancer and adenomas. *Nutr Rev.* 2010 Jul;68(7):389–408.

66   Kesse E, Clavel-Chapelon F, Boutron-Ruault MC. Dietary patterns and risk of colorectal tumors: a cohort of French women of the National Education System (E3N). *Am J Epidemiol.* 2006 Dec 1;164(11):1085–93.

67   Nettleton JA, et al. Meta-analysis investigating associations between healthy diet and fasting glucose and insulin levels and modification by loci associated with glucose homeostasis in data from 15 cohorts. *Am J Epidemiol.* 2013 Jan 15;177(2):103–15.

68   King JC, Slavin JL. White potatoes, human health, and dietary guidance. *Adv Nutr.* 2013 May 1;4(3):S393–401.

69   Storey ML, Anderson PA. Contributions of white vegetables to nutrient intake: NHANES 2009-2010. *Adv Nutr.* 2013 May 1;4(3):S335–44.

70   Weaver C. Potassium and health. *Adv Nutr.* 2013 May 1;4(3):S368–77.

71   Holt SH, Brand Miller JC, Petocz P. An insulin index of foods: the insulin demand generated by 1000-kJ portions of common foods. *Am J Clin Nutr.* 1997 Nov;66(5):1274–76.

72   Holt SH, et al. A satiety index of common foods. *Eur J Clin Nutr.* 1995 Sep;49(9):675–90.

73   Environmental Working Group. "Executive Summary: EWG's 2013 Shopper's Guide to Pesticides in Produce.™" Retrieved from: http://www.ewg.org /foodnews/summary.php. Accessed May 21, 2013.

74   University of Guelph Food Science Network. "Natural Toxins in Fruits and Vegetables." Retrieved from: http://www.uoguelph.ca/foodsafetynetwork /natural-toxins-fruits-and-vegetables. Accessed April 12, 2013.

Chapter 4: Classics!

1   Novotny JA, et al. Discrepancy between the Atwater factor predicted and empirically measured energy value of almonds in human diets. *Am J Clin Nutr.* 2012;96(2):296–301.

2   Morris MC, et al. Vitamin E and cognitive decline in older persons. *Arch Neurol.* 2002 Jul;59(7):1125–32.

3   Wengreen HJ, et al. Antioxidant intake and cognitive function of elderly men and women: the Cache County study. *J Nutr Health Aging.* 2007 May-Jun;11(3):230–7.

4   Martin A, et al. Effects of fruits and vegetables on levels of vitamins E and C in the brain and their association with cognitive performance. *J Nutr Health Aging.* 2002;6(6):392–404.

5   Jenkins DJ, et al. Effects of a dietary portfolio of cholesterol-lowering foods vs lovastatin on serum lipids and C-reactive protein. *JAMA.* 2003 Jul 23:290(4):502–10.

6   Gigleux I, et al. Comparison of a dietary portfolio of cholesterol-lowering foods and a statin on LDL particle size phenotype in hypercholesterolaemic participants. *Br J Nutr.* 2007 Dec;98(6):1229–36.

7   Damasceno NR. Crossover study of diets enriched with virgin olive oil, walnuts or almonds. Effects on lipids and other cardiovascular risk markers. *Nutr Metab Cardiovasc Dis.* 2011 Jun;21 Suppl 1:S14–20.

8   Wien M. Almond consumption and cardiovascular risk factors in adults with prediabetes. *J Am Coll Nutr.* 2010 Jun;29(3):189–97.

9   Cohen AE, Johnston CS. Almond ingestion at mealtime reduces postprandial glycemia and chronic ingestion reduces hemoglobin A(1c) in individuals with well-controlled type 2 diabetes mellitus. *Metabolism.* 2011 Sep;60(9):1312–7.

10   Platt ID, et al. Postprandial effects of almond consumption on human osteoclast precursors—an ex vivo study. *Metabolism.* 2011 Jul;60(7):923–9.

11   Hollis J, Mattes R. Effect of chronic consumption of almonds on body weight in healthy humans. *Br J Nutr.* 2007 Sep;98(3):651–6.

12   California Avocado Commission. "California Avocado History." California avocado.com. Retrieved from: http://www.californiaavocado.com/califor nia-avocado-history. Accessed April 21, 2013.

13   Hass Avocados. "Hass Mother Tree." Avocadocentral.com. Retrieved from: http://www.avocadocentral.com/about-hass-avocados/hass-mother-tree. Accessed May 11, 2013.

14   Fulgoni VL III, Dreher M, Davenport AJ. Avocado consumption is associated

with better diet quality and nutrient intake, and lower metabolic syndrome risk in US adults: results from the National Health and Nutrition Examination Survey (NHANES) 2001–2008. *Nutr J.* 2013 Jan 2;12(1):1.

15 López Ledesma R, et al. Monounsaturated fatty acid (avocado) rich diet for mild hypercholesterolemia. *Arch Med Res.* 1996 Winter;27(4):519–23.

16 Alvizouri-Munoz M, et al. Effects of avocado as a source of monounsaturated fatty acids on plasma lipid levels. *Arch Med Res.* 1992 Winter;23(4):163–7.

17 Lerman-Garber I, et al. Effect of a high-monounsaturated fat diet enriched with avocado in NIDDM patients. *Diabetes Care.* 1994 Apr;17(4):311–5.

18 Dreher ML, Davenport AJ. Hass avocado consumption and potential health benefits. *Crit Rev Food Sci Nutr.* 2013;53(7):738–50.

19 Rosenblat G, et al. Polyhydroxylated fatty alcohols derived from avocado suppress inflammatory response and provide non-sunscreen protection against UV-induced damage in skin cells. *Arch Dermatol Res.* 2011 May;303(4):239–46.

20 Nayak BS, Raju SS, Chalapathi Rao AV. Wound healing activity of *Persea americana* (avocado) fruit: a preclinical study on rats. *J Wound Care.* 2008 Mar;17(3):123–6.

21 American Society for the Prevention of Cruelty to Animals. "Avocado." ASPCA.org. Retrieved from: http://www.aspca.org/pet-care/poison-control/plants/avocado.aspx. Accessed April 21, 2013.

22 Food and Agriculture Organization of the United Nations and World Health Organization. *Codex Alimentarius: Cereals, Pulses, Legumes, and Vegetable Proteins.* First edition. 2007. Retrieved from: ftp://ftp.fao.org/codex/Publications/Booklets/Cereals/CEREALS_2007_EN.pdf. Accessed February 19, 2013.

23 Thompson MD, et al. Mechanisms associated with dose-dependent inhibition of rat mammary carcinogenesis by dry bean (*Phaseolus vulgaris*, L.). *J Nutr.* 2008 Nov;138(11):2091–7.

24 Calderón-Montaño JM, et al. A review on the dietary flavonoid kaempferol. *Mini Rev Med Chem.* 2011 Apr;11(4):298–344.

25 Laparra JM, Glahn RP, Miller DD. Bioaccessibility of phenols in common beans (*Paseolus vulgaris* L.) and iron (Fe) availability to Caco-2 cells. *J Agric Food Chem.* 2008 Nov 26;56(22):10999–1005.

26 Hu Y, et al. Kaempferol in red and pinto bean seed (*Phaseolus vulgaris* L.) coats inhibits iron bioavailability using an in vitro digestion/human Caco-2 cell model. *J Agric Food Chem.* 2006 Nov 29;54(24):9254–61.

27 Pulse News Network, Nutrition Edition. "Pulse Consumption in Canadian Adults Improves Nutrient Intakes." Pulsecanada.com. Retrieved from: http://

www.pulsecanada.com/pnn/nutrition/2012/april/pulse-competition-canadian-adults-improves-intakes-full. Accessed April 23, 2013.

28 Darmadi-Blackberry I, et al. Legumes: the most important dietary predictor of survival in older people of different ethnicities. *Asia Pac J Clin Nutr.* 2004;13(2):217–20.

29 Bazzano LA, et al. Legume consumption and risk of coronary heart disease in US men and women: NHANES I Epidemiologic Follow-up Study. *Arch Intern Med.* 2001 Nov 26;161(21):2573–8.

30 Nöthlings U, et al. Intake of vegetables, legumes, and fruit, and risk for all-cause, cardiovascular, and cancer mortality in a European diabetic population. *J Nutr.* 2008 Apr;138(4):775–81.

31 Abeysekara S, et al. A pulse-based diet is effective for reducing total and LDL-cholesterol in older adults. *Br J Nutr.* 2012 Aug;108 Suppl 1:S103–10.

32 Sievenpiper JL, et al. Effect on non-oil-seed pulses on glycaemic control: a systematic review and meta-analysis of randomised controlled experimental trials in people with and without diabetes. *Diabetologia.* 2009 Aug;52(8):1479–95.

33 Thompson SV, Winham DM, Hutchins AM. Bean and rice meals reduce postprandial glycemic response in adults with type 2 diabetes: a cross-over study. *Nutr J.* 2012 Apr 11;11:23.

34 Kumar S, et al. Phytohemagglutinins augment red kidney bean (*Phaseolus vulgaris* L.) induced allergic manifestations. *J Proteomics.* 2013 Feb 20. [Epub ahead of print.]

35 U.S. Food and Drug Administration. "Phytohaemagglutinin." *Bad Bug Book: Handbook of Foodborne Pathogenic Microorganisms and Natural Toxins.* Retrieved from: http://www.fda.gov/downloads/Food/FoodborneIllness Contaminants/UCM297627.pdf. Accessed April 11, 2013.

36 United Nations Food and Agriculture Organization. "Pulses." *UNFAO/ GIEWS—Food Outlook No. 4.* October 14, 2001. Retrieved from: http://www .fao.org/docrep/005/y6027e/y6027e06.htm. Accessed February 19, 2013.

37 Pollan M. *The Omnivore's Dilemma: A Natural History of Four Meals.* New York: Penguin Press, 2006.

38 Encyclopedia Britannica. "Beet." Britannica.com. Retrieved from: http:// www.britannica.com/EBchecked/topic/58462/beet. Accessed May 19, 2013.

39 Meldrum DR, et al. Lifestyle and metabolic approaches to maximizing erectile and vascular health. *Int J Impot Res.* 2012 Mar-Apr;24(2):61–8.

40 Siervo M, et al. Inorganic nitrate and beetroot juice supplementation reduces blood pressure in adults: a systematic review and meta-analysis. *J Nutr.* 2013 Apr 17. [Epub ahead of print.]

41   Sacks FM, et al. Effects on blood pressure of reduced dietary sodium and the Dietary Approaches to Stop Hypertension (DASH) diet. *N Engl J Med.* 2001;344:3–10.

42   Bailey SJ, et al. The nitrate-nitrite-nitric oxide pathway: its role in human exercise physiology. *Eur J Sport Sci.* 2012;12(4):309–20.

43   Bryan NS, et al. Ingested nitrate and nitrite and stomach cancer risk: an updated review. *Food Chem Toxicol.* 2012 Oct;50(10):3646–65.

44   Jones AM, Bailey SJ, Vanhatalo A. Dietary nitrate and O_2 consumption during exercise. *Med Sport Sci.* 2012;59:29–35.

45   Murphy M, et al. Whole beetroot consumption acutely improves running performance. *J Acad Nutr Diet.* 2012 Apr;112(4):548–52.

46   Hoon MW, et al. The effect of nitrate supplementation on exercise performance in healthy individuals: a systematic review and meta-analysis. *Int J Sport Nutr Exerc Metab.* 2013 Apr 9. [Epub ahead of print]

47   Agriculture and Agri-Food Canada. "A Snapshot of the Canadian Fruit Industry, 2009." Agr.gc.ca. Last modified July 8, 2011. Retrieved from: http://www4 .agr.gc.ca/AAFC-AAC/display-afficher.do?id=1294265926815&lang=eng. Accessed April 25, 2013.

48   Halvorsen BL, et al. Content of redox-active compounds (ie, antioxidants) in foods consumed in the United States. *Am J Clin Nutr.* 2006;84:95–135.

49   Seeram NP, et al. Comparison of antioxidant potency of commonly consumed polyphenol-rich beverages in the United States. *J Agric Food Chem.* 2008;56:1415–22.

50   Cassidy A, et al. High anthocyanin intake is associated with a reduced risk of myocardial infarction in young and middle-aged women. *Circulation.* 2013 Jan;127(2):188–96.

51   Basu A, et al. Blueberries decrease cardiovascular risk factors in obese men and women with metabolic syndrome. *J Nutr.* 2010 Sep;140(9):1582–7.

52   Devore EE, et al. Dietary intakes of berries and flavonoids in relation to cognitive decline. *Ann Neurol.* 2012 Jul;72(1):135–43.

53   Krikorian R, et al. Blueberry supplementation improves memory in older adults. *J Agric Food Chem.* 2010 Apr;58(7):3996–4000.

54   Kay CD, Holub BJ. The effect of wild blueberry (*Vaccinium angustifolium*) consumption on postprandial serum antioxidant status in human subjects. *Br J Nutr.* 2002 Oct;88(4):389–98.

55   McAnulty LS, et al. Effect of blueberry ingestion on natural killer cell counts, oxidative stress, and inflammation prior to and after 2.5 h of running. *Appl Physiol Nutr Metab.* 2011 Dec;36(6):976–84.

56   Clegg ME, et al. The addition of raspberries and blueberries to a starch-based food does not alter the glycaemic response. *Br J Nutr.* 2011 Aug;106(3):335–8.

57   Stull AJ, et al. Bioactives in blueberries improve insulin sensitivity in obese, insulin-resistant men and women. *J Nutr.* 2010; 140:1764–8.

58   Pearson, L. *When in Doubt, Eat Broccoli.* Toronto: Penguin, 1998.

59   Pesticide Risk Reduction Program, Pest Management Centre."Crop Profile for Cabbage and Broccoli in Canada." Agriculture and Agri-Food Canada. 2005. Retrieved from: http://publications.gc.ca/collections/collection_2009/agr /A118-10-9-2005E.pdf. Accessed May 20, 2013.

60   Agriculture and Agri-Food Canada. "A Snapshot of the Canadian Vegetable Industry, 2010." Agr.gc.ca. Last modified March 23, 2012. Retrieved from: http://www4.agr.gc.ca/AAFC-AAC/display-afficher .do?id=1330373416993&lang=eng. Accessed May 21, 2013.

61   Sommerburg O, et al. Fruits and vegetables that are sources for lutein and zeaxanthin: the macular pigment in human eyes. *Br J Opthamol.* 1998 Aug;82(2):907–10.

62   Wu QJ, et al. Cruciferous vegetables intake and the risk of colorectal cancer: a meta-analysis of observational studies. *Ann Oncol.* 2012 Dec 4. [Epub ahead of print.]

63   Steevens J, et al. Vegetables and fruits consumption and risk of esophageal and gastric cancer subtypes in the Netherlands Cohort Study. *Int J Cancer.* 2011 Dec 1;129(11):2681–93.

64   Takahashi K, et al. Effects of total and green vegetable intakes on glycated hemoglobin A1c and triglycerides in elderly patients with type 2 diabetes mellitus: the Japanese Elderly Intervention Trial. *Geriatr Gerontol Int.* 2012 Apr;12 Suppl 1:S50–8.

65   Bahadoran Z, et al. Broccoli sprouts reduce oxidative stress in type 2 diabetes: a randomized double-blind clinical trial. *Eur J Clin Nutr.* 2011 Aug;65(8):972–7.

66   Christiansen B, et al. Ingestion of broccoli sprouts does not improve endo-thelial function in humans with hypertension. *PLoS One.* 2010 Aug 27;5(80):e12461.

67   Fisher JO, et al. Offering "dip" promotes intake of a moderately-liked raw veg-etable among preschoolers with genetic sensitivity to bitterness. *J Acad Nutr Diet.* 2012 Feb;112(2):235–45.

68   Takeda S, et al. Effects of mayonnaise on postprandial serum lutein/zea-xanthin and beta-carotene concentrations in humans. *J Nutr Sci Vitaminol (Tokyo).* 2009 Dec;55(6):479–85.

69   Health Canada. "Caffeine in Food." Retrieved from: http://www.hc-sc .gc.ca/fn-an/securit/addit/caf/food-caf-aliments-eng.php. Accessed March 21, 2013.

70   Gasinska A, Gajewska D. Tea and coffee as the main sources of oxalate in diets of patients with kidney oxalate stones. *Rocz Panstw Zakl Hig.* 2007;58:61–7.

71 Temme EH, Van Hoydonck PG. Tea consumption and iron status. *Eur J Clin Nutr.* 2002 May;56(5):379–86.

72 Jurgens TM, et al. Green tea for weight loss and weight maintenance in overweight and obese adults. *Cochrane Database Syst Rev.* 2012 Dec 12;12:CD008650.

73 Kuriyama S, et al. Green tea consumption and mortality due to cardiovascular disease, cancer, and all causes in Japan: the Ohsaki study. *JAMA.* 2006;296:1255–65.

74 Imai K, Nakachi K. Cross sectional study of effects of drinking green tea on cardiovascular and liver diseases. *BMJ.* 1995;310:693–6.

75 Wang ZM, et al. Black and green tea consumption and the risk of coronary artery disease: a meta-analysis. *Am J Clin Nutr.* 2011 Mar;93(3):506–15.

76 Zheng XX, et al. Green tea intake lowers fasting serum total and LDL cholesterol in adults: a meta-analysis of 14 randomized controlled trials. *Am J Clin Nutr.* 2011 Aug;94(2):601–10.

77 Kim A, et al. Green tea catechins decrease total and low-density lipoprotein cholesterol: a systematic review and meta-analysis. *J Am Diet Assoc.* 2011 Nov;111(11):1720–9.

78 Kempf K, et al. Effects of coffee consumption on subclinical inflammation and other risk factors for type 2 diabetes: a clinical trial. *Am J Clin Nutr.* 2010;91:950–7.

79 Zheng XX, et al. Effects of green tea catechins with or without caffeine on glycemic control in adults: a meta-analysis of randomized controlled trials. *Am J Clin Nutr.* 2013 Apr;97(4):750–62.

80 Zheng J, et al. Green tea and black tea consumption and prostate cancer risk: an exploratory meta-analysis of observational studies. *Nutr Cancer.* 2011; 63(5):663–72.

81 Butler LM, Wu AH. Green and black tea in relation to gynecologic cancers. *Mol Nutr Food Res.* 2011 Jun;55(6):931–40.

82 Fon Sing M, et al. Epidemiological studies of the association between tea drinking and primary liver cancer: a meta-analysis. *Eur J Cancer Prev.* 2011 May;20(3):157–65.

83 Ogunleye AA, Xue F, Michels KB. Green tea consumption and breast cancer risk or recurrence: a meta-analysis. *Breast Cancer Res Treat.* 2010 Jan;119(2):477–84.

84 Egert S, et al. Simultaneous ingestion of dietary proteins reduces the bioavailability of galloylated catechins from green tea in humans. *Eur J Nutr.* 2013 Feb;52(1):281–8.

85 A Dictionary of the English Language. A Digital Edition of the 1755 Classic

by Samuel Johnson. "Oats." Retrieved from: http://johnsonsdictionaryonline
.com/?p=3471. Accessed April 15, 2013.

86   Whole Grains Council. "Oats—January Grain of the Month." Retrieved from:
      http://wholegrainscouncil.org/whole-grains-101/oats-january-grain-of-the
      -month. Accessed April 15, 2013.

87   Othman RA, Moghadasian MH, Jones PJ. Cholesterol-lowering effect of oat
      β-glucan. *Nutr Rev.* 2011 Jun;69(6):299–309.

88   Tiwari U, Cummins E. Meta-analysis of the effect of β-glucan intake on blood
      cholesterol and glucose levels. *Nutrition.* 2011 Oct;27(10):1008–16.

89   Tighe P, et al. Effect of increased consumption of whole-grain foods on blood
      pressure and other cardiovascular risk markers in healthy middle-aged per-
      sons: a randomized controlled trial. *Am J Clin Nutr.* 2010 Oct;92(4):733–40.

90   Sacks FM, et al. Effects on blood pressure of reduced dietary sodium and
      the Dietary Approaches to Stop Hypertension (DASH) diet. *N Engl J Med.*
      2001;344:3–10.

91   Tiwari U, Cummins E. Meta-analysis of the effect of β-glucan intake on blood
      cholesterol and glucose levels. *Nutrition.* 2011 Oct;27(10):1008–16.

92   Lammert A, et al. Clinical benefit of a short term dietary oatmeal intervention
      in patients with type 2 diabetes and severe insulin resistance: a pilot study. *Exp
      Clin Endocrinol Diabetes.* 2008 Feb;116(2):132–4.

93   Chiu CJ, et al. Informing food choices and health outcomes by use of the
      dietary glycemic index. *Nutr Rev.* 2011 Apr;69(4):231–42.

94   Aleem E. β-glucans and their applications in cancer therapy: focus on human
      studies. *Anticancer Agents Med Chem.* 2012 Nov 5. [Epub ahead of print.]

95   Guo W, et al. Avenanthramides inhibit proliferation of human colon cancer
      cell lines in vitro. *Nutr Cancer.* 2010;62(8):1007–16.

96   Fowler JF, et al. Colloidal oatmeal formulations as adjunct treatments in atopic
      dermatitis. *J Drugs Dermatol.* 2012 Jul;11(7):804–7.

97   Virtanen SM, et al. Early introduction of oats associated with decreased risk
      of persistent asthma and early introduction of fish with decreased risk of aller-
      gic rhinitis. *Br J Nutr.* 2010 Jan;103(2):266–73.

98   Nwaru BI, et al. Timing of infant feeding in relation to childhood asthma and
      allergic diseases. *J Allergy Clin Immunol.* 2013 Jan;131(1):78–86.

99   Canadian Celiac Association. "Position Statement on Oats." Retrieved from:
      http://www.celiac.ca/index.php/about-celiac-disease-2/cca-position-state
      ments/position-statement-on-oats. Accessed April 15, 2013.

100   Hanna, S. *The Book of Kale.* Pender Harbour, BC: Harbour Publishing, 2012,
      p. 9.

101 Heaney RP, Weaver CM, Recker RR. Calcium absorbability from spinach. *Am J Clin Nutr.* 1988;47:707–9.

102 Heaney RP, Weaver CM. Calcium absorption from kale. *Am J Clin Nutr.* 1990;51:656–7.

103 Environmental Working Group. "Executive Summary: EWG's 2013 Shopper's Guide to Pesticides in Produce.™" Retrieved from: http://www.ewg.org/foodnews/summary.php. Accessed May 22, 2013.

104 Gijsbers BL, Jie KS, Vermeer C. Effect of food composition on vitamin K absorption in human volunteers. *Br J Nutr.* 1996 Aug;76(2):223–9.

105 Shearer MJ, Fu X, Booth SL. Vitamin K nutrition, metabolism, and requirements: current concepts and future research. *Adv Nutr.* 2012 Mar 1;3(2):182–5.

106 Pan Y, Jackson RT. Dietary phylloquinone intakes and metabolic syndrome in US young adults. *J Am Coll Nutr.* 2009 Aug;28(4):369–79.

107 Yoshida M, et al. Phylloquinone intake, insulin sensitivity, and glycemic status in men and women. *Am J Clin Nutr.* 2008;88:210–5.

108 Braam L, et al. Dietary phylloquinone intake as a potential marker for a heart-healthy dietary pattern in the Framingham Offspring cohort. *J Am Diet Assoc.* 2004 Sep;104(9):1410–4.

109 Juanola-Falgarona M, et al. Association between dietary phylloquinone intake and peripheral metabolic risk markers related to insulin resistance and diabetes in elderly subjects at high cardiovascular risk. *Cardiovasc Diabetol.* 2013 Jan 8;12:7.

110 Hanna S. *The Book of Kale.* Pender Harbour, BC: Harbour Publishing, 2012, p. 9.

111 Agriculture and Agri-Food Canada. "A Snapshot of the Canadian Fruit Industry, 2009." Agr.gc.ca. Last modified July 8, 2011. Retrieved from: http://www4.agr.gc.ca/AAFC-AAC/display-afficher.do?id=1294265926815&lang=eng. Accessed April 25, 2013.

112 University of Sydney. "Glycemic Index: Strawberries, Fresh, Raw." Glycemicindex.com. Last updated June 21, 2012. Retrieved from: http://www.glycemicindex.com/foodSearch.php?num=384&ak=detail. Accessed April 25, 2013.

113 Basu A, et al. Strawberries decrease atherosclerotic markers in subjects with metabolic syndrome. *Nutr Res.* 2010 Jul;30(7):462–9.

114 Jenkins DJ, et al. The effect of strawberries in a cholesterol-lowering dietary portfolio. *Metabolism.* 2008 Dec;57(12):1636–44.

115 Burton-Freeman B. Strawberry modulates LDL oxidation and postprandial lipemia in response to high-fat meal in overweight hyperlipidemic men and women. *J Am Coll Nutr.* 2010 Feb;29(1):46–54.

116 Zunino SJ, et al. Effects of dietary strawberry powder on blood lipids and inflammatory markers in obese human subjects. *Br J Nutr.* 2012 Sep;108(5):900–9.

117 Adhami VM, et al. Dietary flavonoid fisetin: a novel dual inhibitor of PI3K/ Akt and mTOR for prostate cancer treatment. *Biochem Pharmacol.* 2012 Nov;84(10):1277–81.

118 Chen T, et al. Randomized phase II trial of lyophilized strawberries in patients with dysplastic precancerous lesions of the esophagus. *Cancer Prev Res (Phila).* 2012 Jan;5(1):41–50.

119 Environmental Working Group. "Executive Summary: EWG's 2013 Shopper's Guide to Pesticides in Produce.™" Retrieved from: http://www.ewg.org /foodnews/summary.php. Accessed May 21, 2013.

120 Vogt R, et al. Cancer and non-cancer health effects from food contaminant exposures for children and adults in California: a risk assessment. *Environ Health.* 2012 Nov;11:83.

121 Sommerburg O, et al. Fruits and vegetables that are sources for lutein and zeaxanthin: the macular pigment in human eyes. *Br J Ophthamol.* 1998;82:907–910.

122 Gleize B, et al. Effect of type of TAG fatty acids on lutein and zeaxanthin bioavailability. *Br J Nutr.* 2012;Dec 11:1–10. [Epub ahead of print.]

123 Heaney RP, Weaver CM, Recker RR. Calcium absorbability from spinach. *Am J Clin Nutr.* 1988;47:707–9.

124 Faith NG, Waldron T, Czuprynski CJ. Reduction in resident microflora, and experimentally inoculated Salmonella enterica, on spinach leaves treated with vinegar and canola oil. *J Food Prot.* 2012 Mar;75(3):567–72.

125 Siervo M, et al. Inorganic nitrate and beetroot juice supplementation reduces blood pressure in adults: a systematic review and meta-analysis. *J Nutr.* 2013 Apr 17. [Epub ahead of print.]

126 Bailey SJ, et al. The nitrate-nitrite-nitric oxide pathway: its role in human exercise physiology. *Eur J Sport Sci.* 2012 July;12(4):309–20.

127 Bondonno CP, et al. Flavonoid-rich apples and nitrate-rich spinach augment nitric oxide status and improve endothelial function in healthy men and women: a randomized controlled trial. *Free Radic Biol Med.* 2012 Jan 1;52(1):95–102.

128 Johnson M, Pace RD. Sweet potato leaves: properties and synergistic interactions that promote health and prevent disease. *Nutr Rev.* 2010 Oct;68(10):604–15.

129 Agriculture and Agri-Food Canada. "A Snapshot of the Canadian Vegetable Industry, 2010." Agr.gc.ca. Last modified March 23, 2012. Retrieved from: http://www4

.agr.gc.ca/AAFC-AAC/display-afficher.do?id=1330373416993&lang=eng. Accessed May 21, 2013.

130 Mills JP, et al. Sweet potato beta-carotene bioefficacy is enhanced by dietary fat and not reduced by soluble fiber intake in Mongolian gerbils. *J Nutr.* 2009 Jan;139(1):44–50.

131 Ludvik B, Neuffer B, Pacini G. Efficacy of *Ipomoea batatas* (Caiapo) on diabetes control in type 2 diabetic subjects treated with diet. *Diabetes Care.* 2004 Feb;27(2):436–40.

132 Ludvik B, et al. Mode of action of *Ipomoea batatas* (Caiapo) in type 2 diabetic patients. *Metabolism.* 2003 Jul;52(7):875–80.

133 Ludvik BH, et al. The effect of *Ipomoea batatas* (Caiapo) on glucose metabolism and serum cholesterol in patients with type 2 diabetes: a randomized study. *Diabetes Care.* 2002 Jan;25(1):239–40.

134 Ooi CP, Loke SC. Sweet potato for type 2 diabetes mellitus. *Cochrane Database Syst Rev.* 2012 Feb 15;2:CD009128.

135 University of Sydney. "Sweet potato." Glycemicindex.com. Last updated June 12, 2012. Retrieved from: http://www.glycemicindex.com/foodSearch.php. Accessed May 16, 2013.

136 Appel LJ, et al. A clinical trial of the effects of dietary patterns on blood pressure. *N Engl J Med.* 1997 Apr;336:1117–24.

137 Al-Okbi SY. Nutraceuticals of anti-inflammatory activity as complementary therapy for rheumatoid arthritis. *Toxicol Ind Health.* 2012 Oct 26. [Epub ahead of print.]

138 Halvorsen BL, et al. Content of redox-active compounds (ie antioxidants) in foods consumed in the United States. *Am J Clin Nutr.* 2006 Jul;84(1): 95–135.

139 Estruch R, et al. Primary prevention of cardiovascular disease with a Mediterranean diet. *N Engl J Med.* 2013 Apr 4;368(14):1279–90.

140 Ros E, et al. A walnut diet improves endothelial function in hypercholesterolemic subjects: a randomized crossover trial. *Circulation.* 2004 Apr 6;109(13):1609–14.

141 Muñoz S, et al. Walnut-enriched diet increases the association of LDL from hypercholesterolemic men with human HepG2 cells. *J Lipid Res.* 2001 Dec;42(12):2069–76.

142 Iwamoto M, et al. Serum lipid profiles in Japanese women and men during consumption of walnuts. *Eur J Clin Nutr.* 2002 Jul;56(7):629–37.

143 Rajaram S, et al. Walnuts and fatty fish influence different serum lipid fractions in normal to mildly hyperlipidemic individuals: a randomized controlled study. *Am J Clin Nutr.* 2009 May;89(5):S1657–63.

144 Haider S, et al. Effects of walnuts (*Juglans regia*) on learning and memory functions. *Plant Foods Hum Nutr.* 2011 Nov;66(4):335–40.

145 Valls-Pedret C, et al. Polyphenol-rich foods in the Mediterranean diet are associated with better cognitive function in elderly subjects at high cardiovascular risk. *J Alzheimers Dis.* 2012;29(4):773–82.

146 Pribis P, et al. Effects of walnut consumption on cognitive performance in young adults. *Br J Nutr.* 2011 Sep 19:1–9.

147 Sabaté J. Nut consumption and body weight. *Am J Clin Nutr.* 2003 Sep;78(3 Suppl):S647–50.

148 Brennan AM, et al. Walnut consumption increases satiation but has no effect on insulin resistance or the metabolic profile over a 4-day period. *Obesity (Silver Spring).* 2010 Jun;18(6):1176–82.

149 Burton-Freeman B. Sex and cognitive dietary restraint influence cholecystokinin release and satiety in response to preloads varying in fatty acid composition and content. *J Nutr.* 2005 Jun;135(6):1407–14.

Chapter 5: Send Me a Hero

1 Macharia-Mutie CW, et al. Maize porridge enriched with a micronutrient powder containing low-dose iron as NaFeEDTA but not amaranth grain flour reduces anemia and iron deficiency in Kenyan preschool children. *J Nutr.* 2012 Sep;142(9):1756–63.

2 Capriles VD, et al. Effects of processing methods on amaranth starch digestibility and predicted glycemic index. *J Food Sci.* 2008 Sep;73(7):H160–4.

3 Qureshi AA, Lehmann JW, Peterson DM. Amaranth and its oil inhibit cholesterol biosynthesis in 6-week-old female chickens. *J Nutr.* 1996 Aug;126(8):1972–8.

4 Berger A, et al. Cholesterol-lowering properties of amaranth grain and oil in hamsters. *Int J Vitam Nutr Res.* 2003 Feb;73(1):39–47.

5 Kim HK, Kim MJ, Shin DH. Improvement of lipid profile by amaranth (*Amaranthus esculantus*) supplementation in streptozotocin-induced diabetic rats. *Ann Nutr Metab.* 2006;50(3):277–81.

6 Caselato-Sousa VM, Amaya-Farfán J. State of knowledge on amaranth grain: a comprehensive review. *J Food Sci.* 2012 Apr;77(4):R93–104.

7 Yang Y, et al. Favorite foods of older adults living in the Black Belt Region of the United States. Influences of ethnicity, gender, and education. *Appetite.* 2013 Apr;63:18–23.

8 Bell KI, Tepper BJ. Short-term vegetable intake by young children classified by 6-n-propylthiouracil bitter-taste phenotype. *Am J Clin Nutr.* 2006 Jul;84(1):245–51.

9   Tordoff MG, Sandell MA. Vegetable bitterness is related to calcium content. *Appetite.* 2009 Apr;52(2):498–504.

10   Gueguen L, Pointillart A. The bioavailability of dietary calcium. *J Am Coll Nutr.* 2000 Apr;19(2 Suppl):S119–36.

11   Lin LZ, Harnly JM. Identification of the phenolic components of collard greens, kale, and Chinese broccoli. *J Agric Food Chem.* 2009 Aug 26;57(16):7401–8.

12   Giaconi JA, et al. The association of consumption of fruits/vegetables with decreased risk of glaucoma among older African-American women in the study of osteoporotic fractures. *Am J Ophthalmol.* 2012 Oct;154(4):635–44.

13   Coleman AL, et al. Glaucoma risk and the consumption of fruits and vegetables among older women in the study of osteoporotic fractures. *Am J Ophthalmol.* 2008 Jun;145(6):1081–9.

14   Kahlon TS, et al. Steam cooking significantly improves in vitro bile acid binding of collard greens, kale, mustard greens, broccoli, green bell pepper, and cabbage. *Nutr Res.* 2008 Jun;28(6):351–7.

15   Kristal AR, Lampe JW. *Brassica* vegetables and prostate cancer risk: a review of the epidemiological evidence. *Nutr Cancer.* 2002;42(1):1–9.

16   Kim MK, Park JH. Conference on "Multidisciplinary approaches to nutritional problems." Symposium on "Nutrition and health." Cruciferous vegetable intake and the risk of human cancer: epidemiological evidence. *Proc Nutr Soc.* 2009 Feb;68(1):103–10.

17   Aune D, et al. Dietary compared with blood concentrations of carotenoids and breast cancer risk: a systematic review and meta-analysis of prospective studies. *Am J Clin Nutr.* 2012 Aug;96(2):356–73.

18   Agriculture and Agri-Food Canada. "A Snapshot of the Canadian Fruit Industry, 2009." Agr.gc.ca. Last modified July 8, 2011. Retrieved from: http://www4 .agr.gc.ca/AAFC-AAC/display-afficher.do?id=1294265926815&lang=eng. Accessed April 23, 2013.

19   California Kiwifruit. "Slooping the Kiwi." Retrieved from: http://www.kiwi fruit.org/about/slooping.aspx. Accessed April 23, 2013.

20   Sommerburg O, et al. Fruits and vegetables that are sources for lutein and zeaxanthin: the macular pigment in human eyes. *Br J Ophthalmol.* 1998;82:907–10.

21   Duttaroy AK, Jorgensen A. Effects of kiwi fruit consumption on platelet aggregation and plasma lipids in healthy human volunteers. *Platelets.* 2004 Aug;15(5):287–92.

22   Chang WH, Liu JF. Effects of kiwifruit consumption on serum lipid profiles

and antioxidative status in hyperlipidemic subjects. *Int J Food Sci Nutr.* 2009 Dec;60(8):709–16.

23   Gammon CS, et al. Kiwifruit consumption favourably affects plasma lipids in a randomised controlled trial in hypercholesterolaemic men. *Br J Nutr.* 2012 Nov;14:1–11.

24   Brevik A, et al. Supplementation of a Western diet with golden kiwifruits (*Actinidia chinensis* var.'Hort 16A':) effects on biomarkers of oxidation damage and antioxidant protection. *Nutr J.* 2011 May 18;10:54.

25   Collins BH, et al. Kiwifruit protects against oxidative DNA damage in human cells and in vitro. *Nutr Cancer.* 2001;39(1):148–52.

26   Chang CC, et al. Kiwifruit improves bowel function in patients with irritable bowel syndrome with constipation. *Asia Pac J Clin Nutr.* 2010;19(4):451–7.

27   Chan AO, et al. Increasing dietary fiber intake in terms of kiwifruit improves constipation in Chinese patients. *World J Gastroenterol.* 2007 Sep 21;13(35):4771–5.

28   Rush EC, et al. Kiwifruit promotes laxation in the elderly. *Asia Pac J Clin Nutr.* 2002;11(2):164–8.

29   Deters AM, Schroder KR, Hensel A. Kiwi fruit (*Actinidia chinensis* L.) polysaccharides exert stimulating effects on cell proliferation via enhanced growth factor receptors, energy production, and collagen synthesis of human keratinocytes, fibroblasts, and skin equivalents. *J Cell Physiol.* 2005 Mar;202(3):717–22.

30   Childs MT, et al. Effects of shellfish consumption on lipoproteins in normolipidemic men. *Am J Clin Nutr.* 1990 Jun;51(6):1020–7.

31   Childs MT, et al. Effect of shellfish consumption on cholesterol absorption on normolipidemic men. *Metabolism.* 1987 Jan;36(1):31–5.

32   Cassady BA, et al. Effects of low carbohydrate diets high in red meats or poultry, fish and shellfish on plasma lipids and weight loss. *Nutr Metab (Lond).* 2007 Oct 31;4:23.

33   Monterey Bay Aquarium Seafood Watch. "Oysters." Retrieved from http://www.seafoodwatch.org/cr/seafoodwatch/web/sfw_factsheet.aspx?fid=82. Accessed December 2, 2013.

34   Monterey Bay Aquarium Seafood Watch. "Mussels." Retrieved from http://www.montereybayaquarium.org//cr/SeafoodWatch/web/sfw_factsheet.aspx?gid=36. Accessed December 2, 2013.

35   Pistachio Health Institute. "Pistachio Fun Facts." Pistachiohealthinstitute.com. Retrieved from: http://www.pistachiohealth.com/consumer/about-pistachios/fun-facts. Accessed March 20, 2013.

36   Instructables. "How to Open a Pesky Pistachio Nut." Instructables.com. Retrieved from: http://www.instructables.com/id/How-To-Open-a-Pesky-Pistachio-Nut. Accessed March 20, 2013.

37   Gebauer SK, et al. Effects of pistachios on cardiovascular disease risk factors and potential mechanisms of action: a dose-response study. *Am J Clin Nutr.* 2008 Sep;88(3):651–9.

38   Sheridan MJ, et al. Pistachio nut consumption and serum lipid levels. *J Am Coll Nutr.* 2007 Apr;26(2):141–8.

39   Kocyigit A, Koylu AA, Keles H. Effects of pistachio nuts consumption on plasma lipid profile and oxidative status in healthy volunteers. *Nutr Metab Cardiovasc Dis.* 2006 Apr;16(3):202–9.

40   Aksoy N, et al. Pistachio intake increases high density lipoprotein levels and inhibits low-density lipoprotein oxidation in rats. *Tohoku J Exp Med.* 2007 May;212(1):43–8.

41   Li Z, et al. Pistachio nuts reduce triglycerides and body weight by comparison to refined carbohydrate snack in obese subjects on a 12-week weight loss program. *J Am Coll Nutr.* 2010 Jun;29(3):198–203.

42   Wang X, et al. Effects of pistachios on body weight in Chinese subjects with metabolic syndrome. *Nutr J.* 2012 Apr 3;11:20.

43   Kendall CW, et al. The impact of pistachio intake alone or in combination with high-carbohydrate foods on post-prandial glycemia. *Eur J Clin Nutr.* 2011 Jun;65(6):696–702.

44   Zaineddin AK, et al. The association between dietary lignans, phytoestrogen-rich foods, and fiber intake and postmenopausal breast cancer risk: a German case-control study. *Nutr Cancer.* 2012;64(5):652–65.

45   Gossell-Williams M, et al. Improvement in HDL cholesterol in postmenopausal women supplemented with pumpkin seed oil: pilot study. *Climacteric.* 2011 Oct;14(5):558–64.

46   Naghii MR, Mofid M. Impact of daily consumption of iron fortified ready-to-eat cereal and pumpkin seed kernels (*Cucurbita pepo*) on serum iron in adult women. *Biofactors.* 2007;30(1):19–26.

47   Health Canada. "Sesame—One of the ten priority food allergens." Last modified October 26, 2012. Retrieved from: http://www.hc-sc.gc.ca/fn-an/pubs/securit/2012-allergen_sesame/index-eng.php. Accessed May 16, 2013.

48   Wu JH, et al. Sesame supplementation does not improve cardiovascular disease risk markers in overweight men and women. *Nutr Metab Cardiovasc Dis.* 2009 Dec;19(11):774–80.

49 Wu WH, et al. Sesame ingestion affects sex hormones, antioxidant status, and blood lipids in postmenopausal women. *J Nutr.* 2006 May;136(5):1270–5.

50 Peterson J, et al. Dietary lignans: physiology and potential for cardiovascular disease risk reduction. *Nutr Rev.* 2010 Oct;68(10):571–603.

INDEX

A

açaí (*Euterpe oleracea*), 6–13
ACE (angiotensin-converting
    enzyme), 37–38
acetylcholine, 101
acrylamide, 119
agave nectar (*Agave tequilana*),
    67–71
  side effects, 70
AgriSalba Corporation, 29
ALA (alpha-linolenic acid), 32,
    48–49, 103, 201. *See also*
    omega-3 fatty acids
allergic reactions, 18, 115–16,
    138, 234
Alliance for Potato Research and
    Education, 120
almonds (*Prunis dulcis*), 124–32
  nutritional profile, 125–27,
    226
Alzheimer's disease, 57
amaranth, 207–10
  nutritional profile, 172, 173,
    208–9, 238
American Diabetes Association,
    130–31
amino acids, 15, 149–50, 209, 231
  in quinoa, 42, 43
Ancient Naturals (Core
    Naturals), 28–30
anthocyanins, 10, 141, 155,
    194–95
anticoagulants, 18, 181, 182
antioxidants, 9–11, 17, 141–42,
    153–54, 201, 217

apoB (apolipoprotein B), 227
appetite control, 32, 39, 131–32,
    205
aquaculture, 222–23
arthritis, 122
asthma, 177
athletic performance, 21, 39, 51,
    157
  coconut water and, 23,
    24–25
  nitric oxide and, 149–51
Atwater, Wilbur Olin, 125
avenanthramides, 176
Aviram, Michael, 37–38
avocado (*Persea americana*),
    132–39
  nutritional profile, 134–35,
    184
  safety concerns, 138

B

bacteria. *See also* salmonella
  in cheese, 88, 90
  and nitrite, 150, 193
  sesame oil and, 234
beans, 145. *See also* pulses
  black, 136, 140, 141–42
  red kidney, 136, 140–42,
    145
  safety concerns, 145
  white kidney, 142, 145
beef, 78–87
beets (*Beta vulgaris*), 147–51
beeturia, 151

beta-carotene, 163, 225
beta-glucan, 172–73
biofuels, 70
blackberries, 154
blinding (of studies), 108, 161
blood clotting, 182–83
blood pressure
    beets and, 148–49
    blueberries and, 155–56
    broccoli and, 162
    cocoa and, 96–97
    oats and, 174–75
    pomegranate juice and, 37–38
    Salba and, 32
    sweet potatoes and, 197–99
blood sugar
    agave nectar and, 70
    blueberries and, 157–58
    broccoli and, 160
    carbohydrates and, 114,
        117–18
    green tea and, 167–68
    nuts and, 130–31, 228–29
    oats and, 175, 176
    pomegranate juice and, 38–39
    potatoes and, 120–21
    pulses and, 144
    seeds and, 32, 209
    sweet potatoes and, 196–97
    vitamin K and, 184–85
blood-thinners, 18, 181, 182
blueberries (*Vaccinium*
    angustifolium), 152–58
    cultivated, 152–53, 154, 158,
        184

nutritional profile, 153–54,
    184
Bolivia, 45–46, 47
bone health, 91, 131, 183
The Book of Kale (Hanna), 179
bowel health, 75, 217–18
brain health, 156–57, 204–5
Brassica family (cruciferous
    vegetables), 160
    broccoli, 158–63
    collard greens, 211–14
    kale, 179–86
breast cancer, 232
broccoli (*Brassica oleracea v.
    italica*), 158–63
    nutritional profile, 159–60,
        184, 196
Brown, Lawrence (Larry), 29
Brown, Thelma, 29
Burnbrae Farms, 102, 103

C

caffeine, 167, 169
    in cocoa and chocolate, 94,
        95
    in coffee, 168
    in tea, 164, 168
calcitonin, 91
calcium, 238
    in almonds, 126–27
    in kale, 180–81, 238
    in seeds, 31, 49, 208, 235, 238
    vitamins and, 91–92
calories, 125–26

cancer, 160. *See also specific types of
   cancer*
   beef and, 83–84
   chemotherapy for, 76
   collard greens and, 213
   green tea and, 168–70
   kiwi and, 217
   oats and, 176–77
   pumpkin seeds and, 232
   strawberries and, 189–90
   vitamin K_2 and, 92
carbohydrates, 24, 80–81, 114,
   209
carboxylation, 183
cardiovascular disease. *See also*
   heart health; plaque
   beef and, 80–83
   broccoli and, 162
   cocoa and, 97–98
   diet and, 129
   eggs and, 105
   green tea and, 166–67
   hemp hearts and, 55
   pomegranate juice and, 37–38
   pulses and, 143–44
carotenoids, 213
Carver, George Washington,
   110–11
catechins, 164
celiac disease, 43, 49
Cerophyl, 72
cheese, 87–93
   eating, 88, 92
chia seeds, 27, 47–52
   nutritional profile, 48–49, 238

chickpeas, 136, 141. *See also* pulses
chocolate, 95, 98–99. *See also*
   cocoa
cholecystokinin, 205
cholesterol. *See also* cholesterol
   control
   caffeine and, 167
   carbohydrates and, 80–81
   and diabetes, 107
   in eggs, 101–2, 106–7
   and heart disease, 107–9
   LDL (damage to), 162
   research on, 129–30
cholesterol control
   agave nectar and, 68–69
   avocado and, 136–37
   cocoa and, 97–98
   coconut and, 64–65
   collard greens and, 213
   diet for, 128–30
   eggs and, 105
   fruits and, 37, 188–89,
      216–17
   grains and, 76, 172–74
   green tea and, 166–67
   medications for, 174, 213
   MUFAs and, 137
   nuts and, 130, 203–4, 225–27,
      229
   oysters and, 222
   peanut butter and, 113–14
   pulses and, 144
   seeds and, 49–50, 57, 236–37
   cholestyramine (Questran),
      213

choline, 101

cocoa (*Theobroma cacao*), 93–99, 168

coconut (*Cocos nucifera*), 59–67. *See also* coconut oil; coconut water

coconut oil, 59, 61–62

coconut water, 22–26

cohort studies, 142–43

cola, 168

collagen, 218

collard greens (*Brassica oleracea v. acephala*), 211–14

    nutritional profile, 184, 196, 212

colorectal cancer, 92, 160, 176

confirmation bias, 108

constipation, 217–18

copper, 94–95, 201, 220, 226

Coumadin (warfarin), 182–83

C-reactive protein (CRP), 129

crossover studies, 106

cytokines, 185

D

dairy products, 89–92. *See also* cheese

DASH diet, 175, 197–99

developing countries, 146, 210

DHA (docosahexaenoic acid), 32, 48, 103, 220–21. *See also* omega-3 fatty acids

diabetes, 70, 82, 137

    eggs and, 104, 105, 106–7

diets, 97. *See also specific foods*

    DASH, 175, 197–99

    for diabetics, 130–31

    and heart health, 113–14, 128–30

    lower-carbohydrate, higher-protein, 106–7

    Mediterranean, 202

    NCEP Step II, 113–14, 128–30

    portfolio, 128–30, 188

    vegetarian, 128, 233

The Dr. Oz Show, 13

E

eczema (atopic dermatitis), 57–58, 177

eggs, 100–109

    omega-3, 102–3, 127

    and salmonella, 104

elderly people, 86

Elvehjem, C.A., 74

endothelial function, 98

end points, 36–37

enterolactone, 236

Environmental Working Group Dirty Dozen list, 122, 181, 190

EPA (eicosapentaenoic acid), 48, 220–21. *See also* omega-3 fatty acids

epigallocatechin gallate (EGCG), 164

erectile dysfunction, 98, 148, 229

European Prospective Investigation into Cancer and Nutrition (EPIC), 144

eye health, 17, 101, 212. *See also* lutein; zeaxanthin

F

FAO (UN Food and Agriculture Organization), 42, 139

fats. *See also* MUFAs; omega-3/-6 fatty acids; PUFAs
  in diet, 113–14
  in foods, 79, 135, 201
  and heart disease, 89–92
  saturated, 61–62, 81
  and vitamin K, 181

FDA (US Food and Drug Administration), 10, 14–15, 34

fibre, 144
  insoluble, 30, 237
  introducing in diet, 27–28
  soluble, 128, 172–73

fisetin, 189

fish oils, 103, 204

flavanols, 98, 99

flavonols, 164

flaxseed, 102–3, 236

folate, 135

food poisoning, 104, 193

foods. *See also* superfoods; *specific foods*
  bitter, 162–63

cooking, 240
  whole, 2, 239–40

Framingham Offspring Study, 184–85

Framingham Risk Score, 173–74

FreeLife International, 14–15

fructans, 69

fructose, 67–68, 69

FTC (US Federal Trade Commission), 34, 35

G

gamma-tocopherol (vitamin E), 225

Gatorade, 23

GLA (gamma-linoleic acid), 54, 58

glaucoma, 212

glucosinolates, 212, 213

glutathione peroxidase (GSH-Px), 17

gluten, 43, 49, 178

glycemic index (GI)
  of agave nectar, 67–68
  of amaranth, 209
  of oats, 176
  of potatoes, 121
  of pulses, 144
  of quinoa, 44
  of strawberries, 187
  of sweet potatoes, 197

GoChi Juice, 15, 16–17

goji berries (*Lycium barbarum, L. chinense*), 13–18
  nutritional profile, 15–16, 196

goji berries (*cont.*)
  side effects, 18
Gordon, Ben, 13
grains, 173. *See also specific grains
  and pseudograins*

H

Hanna, Sharon, 179
Harpo, Inc., 13
Hass, Rudolph, 133
Health, Aging and Body
    Composition (Health
    ABC) study, 105, 107
Health Professionals Follow-Up
    Study, 103–4
Heaney, Robert, 181
heart health. *See also* blood
    pressure; cardiovascular
    disease; cholesterol control
  avocado and, 135–37
  beef and, 80–83
  berries and, 7, 21, 155–56,
    188–89
  cholesterol and, 107–9
  coconut and, 63–65
  diet and, 113–14, 128–30
  eggs and, 103–4
  fats and, 81, 111
  kiwi and, 216–17
  magnesium and, 55
  nuts and, 113–15, 202–4,
    225–27
  oysters and mussels and,
    221–22

pulses and, 144
  seeds and, 32, 50, 57, 232,
    236–37
  studies of, 127–30
  vitamins and, 90–91, 143
Heinicke, Ralph, 18
hemp hearts, 52–59
hemp oil, 57–58
hormones, 237
Hu, Frank, 107
hyponatremia, 25

I

IBS (irritable bowel syndrome),
    218
inflammation, 185, 199, 213
insulin, 121. *See also* blood sugar;
    diabetes
  carbohydrates and, 114
  pomegranate juice and, 37–38
  potatoes and, 121–22
  resistance to, 117
  sensitivity to, 37–38, 130–31,
    184–85
inulin, 69
iron
  in beans, 142
  in beef, 79–80, 83
  pumpkin seeds and, 232–33
  in seeds, 31, 208, 231, 235
  wheat grass and, 75–76
Isner, John, 25

J

Jenkins, David, 100, 127–31, 228–29
Jeremiah, Stefan, 46
Joseph Enterprises, 47

K

kaempferol, 142, 212
kale (*Brassica oleracea v. acephala*), 179–86
   eating, 180, 181, 185
   nutritional profile, 179–81, 184, 196, 238
kiwi fruit (*Actinidia polygama*), 214–19
   golden (*A. chinensis*), 217
   nutritional profile, 184, 215–16
Kohler, George C., 74
Kris-Etherton, Penny, 113–14
Kuna Indians, 96

L

Lacto-Wolfberry, 17
lauric acid, 61–62
LCFAs (long-chain fatty acids), 62
lectins, 145
legumes. *See* pulses
lentils, 136, 140, 141, 144. *See also* pulses
lignans, 236–37
lignins, 237

linoleic acid. *See* omega-6 fatty acids
lipids, 225–27. *See also* cholesterol; triglycerides
lovastatin, 128–30
lutein, 101, 163, 192–93, 216, 225
lysine, 209

M

macular degeneration. *See* eye health
magnesium, 195
   in nuts, 126, 201
   in seeds, 31, 55, 208, 231–32
manganese, 55, 221
mangel-wurzels (mangolds), 147
Manitoba Harvest Hemp Foods, 54, 58
Manson, JoAnn, 107
McCallum, E.Y., 74–75
Mealla, Adolfo and Alfredo, 27, 29–30, 32
meat. *See also* beef
   cooking, 83, 84
   grass-fed, 82
   processing of, 81–82
   serving sizes, 86–87
memory, 204–5
menopause, 57, 237
meta-analysis, 97
metabolic syndrome, 50, 136–37, 184–85, 228
MGP (matrix Gla-protein), 91
MonaVie LLC, 7, 11, 13

Monterey Bay Aquarium, 222–23

Morinda Bioactives, 19, 20, 21

mortality, 143

The Mother Grain (Jeremiah and Wilcox), 46

MUFAs (monounsaturated fats), 113–14, 137, 225

multi-level marketing (MLM), 13, 14, 20

muscles, 84–87

mussels, 219–23

myristic acid, 61–62

N

National Cholesterol Education Program (NCEP) Step II diet, 113–14, 128–30

National Health and Nutrition Examination Survey (NHANES), 120, 135–37

Follow-Up Study, 143–44

natto, 182

Naturegg Omega Pro eggs, 102, 103

Navitas Naturals, 14, 15

The Newer Knowledge of Nutrition (McCallum), 74–75

nightshade family, 122

nitrates, 84, 148–51

nitric oxide (NO), 21, 98, 148–51

nitrite (NO_2), 150

nitrogen fixation, 146

noni juice (*Morinda citrifolia* L.), 18–21

side effects, 21

Nurses' Health Study, 103–4, 155, 156

nuts, 109–10, 125–26, 226. *See also specific types of nuts*

O

oats (*Avena sativa*), 171–78

olive oil, 113–14

omega-3 fatty acids

eggs containing, 102–3, 127

from seafood, 220–21, 222

in seeds, 31–32, 48–49, 54

in walnuts, 201, 204

omega-6 fatty acids, 56, 225

in seeds, 49, 54, 235

OmniHeart Trial, 81

The Omnivore's Dilemma (Pollan), 82

O.N.E. Coconut Water, 23, 25, 26

The Oprah Winfrey Show, 7, 13

ORAC (oxygen radical absorbance capacity), 10–11

oral immunotherapy (OIT), 115–16

osteoblasts, 183

osteocalcin, 183, 185

osteoclasts, 131, 183

osteoporosis, 183

oxalates, 160, 164, 193, 212

oxidation, 9–10. *See also* antioxidants
oxidative stress, 50, 157
oysters, 219–23
Oz, Mehmet (Dr. Oz), 7, 13–14

P

Paddon-Jones, Douglas, 86
pain (chronic), 122
peanut butter, 109–17
peanuts (*Arachis hypogaea*), 110–11, 112, 115
Pearson, Liz, 158
pepitas. *See* pumpkin seeds
Perricone, Nicholas, 7
pesticides, 122, 181, 190
phenolics, 212
photosensitivity, 18
Physicians' Health Study, 105
phytates, 208
phytoestrogens, 232
phytohemagglutinin (PHA), 145
PINES International, 72–73
pistachios (*Pistacia vera*), 223–30
placebo effect, 161. *See also* blinding
plaque (arterial), 37, 216
Pollan, Michael, 82
polyphenols, 9, 10, 163, 164
pomegranates (*Punica granatum*), 33–40
  nutritional profile, 35, 184
POM Wonderful, 33, 34–35, 36, 37

population studies, 83–84, 142–43, 169
portfolio diet, 128–30, 188
potassium, 136
  in avocado, 135, 136
  in coconut water, 23, 136
  in nuts, 126, 136
  in potatoes, 120, 136
  in seeds, 31, 136
  in sweet potatoes, 136, 195–96, 197–98
potatoes (*Solanum tuberosum*), 117–23
  safety concerns, 122–23
Powerade, 23
PREDIMED (Prevención con Dieta Mediterránea) study, 202–3, 204–5
Prior, Ian, 62–63
Propster, Mitchell A., 29
prostate cancer, 92
protein, 85–87, 129, 231, 233
pseudograins, 173. *See also* amaranth; quinoa
PUFAs (polyunsaturated fatty acids), 48–49. *See also* omega-3/-6 fatty acids
Pukapuka people, 62–63
pulses, 110–11, 139–47
  safety concerns, 145
pumpkin seeds (*Cucurbita*), 230–33
  nutritional profile, 184, 231–32

Q

quercetin, 212
quinoa, 42–47
   nutritional profile, 43, 172,
      173

R

Ralston, William A. and Richard
      L., 28–29
raspberries, 154
Resnick, Lynda and Stewart, 34
rhabdomyolysis, 12

S

Sacks, Frank, 37
Salba Corp., 28–29
Salba Research and
      Development Inc., 29
Salba (*Salvia hispanica* L.), 26–33
   claims about, 26–27, 31–32
   nutritional profile, 30–32, 238
Salba Smart Natural Products,
      28–29
salmon, 219
salmonella, 104, 193
Sambazon, 9
sarcopenia, 85, 86
saturated fats, 61–62, 81, 101
Schnabel, Charles F., 71–72
seafood. *See* mussels; oysters
Seafood Watch, 222–23
Sears, Barry, 106
selenium, 221

sesame seeds (*Sesamum indicum*),
      233–38
sesamin, 236
shellfish. *See* mussels; oysters
skin health, 57–58, 138, 177, 218
sodium, 25, 175
SOD (superoxide dismutase), 17
solanine, 122–23
soybeans, 110–11
spinach (*Spinacia oleracea*), 160,
      191–94
   nutritional profile, 184, 191–
      93, 196
sports drinks. *See* athletic
      performance
squalene, 210
starches. *See* carbohydrates
statins, 128–30
stomach cancer, 160
strawberries (*Fragaria* x *ananassa*),
      186–90
   nutritional profile, 154, 187
studies. *See also specific studies*
   blinded, 108, 161
   cohort, 142–43
   confirmation bias in, 108
   controlled, 108, 161
   crossover, 106
   meta-analysis, 97
   population, 83–84, 142–43,
      169
   powdered foods in, 157, 161–
      62, 189–90
   prospective, 202
   retrospective, 169

sugar beets, 147
superfoods, 1–3
  as fads, 5–6, 239
  marketing scams, 13, 14, 20
  trademark issues, 27, 28–30
  unfounded claims, 13, 26,
    34–35
supplements, 72–73
surrogate markers, 36–37
sweet potatoes (*Ipomoea batatas*),
  194–200
Swiss chard (leaf beets), 147,
  160

T

Tahitian Noni, 19, 20, 21
tea, 163, 168
  green (*Camellia sinensis*),
    163–70
thalassemia, 75
thermogenesis, 165
Tokelau people, 62–63
triglycerides, 68–69, 81, 114, 160,
  216–17, 222
  medium-chain (MCTs),
    61–62

U

ulcerative colitis, 75
United States Department of
  Agriculture (USDA), 10, 53

V

vasodilation, 98, 148, 193
vegetarians, 84, 105, 128
  nutrition sources, 52, 55, 233
Vita Coco, 23, 25–26
vitamin A, 196
  in broccoli, 159–60, 196
  in goji berries, 15–16, 196
  in kale, 180, 196
  in sweet potatoes, 195, 196
B vitamins, 135, 180, 195, 224–25,
  235
  in oysters and mussels (B_{12}),
    220, 221
vitamin C, 159, 180, 187, 195,
  215
vitamin D
  and calcium, 91–92
  and heart disease, 143
vitamin E, 126, 127, 225
  in kiwi, 127, 215
  in pistachios, 225
vitamin K, 159, 180, 181, 215
  menaquinone (K_2), 90–92,
    182
  phylloquinone (K_1), 90–91,
    182–85
Vuksan, Vladimir, 27, 32

W

walnuts (*Juglans regia*), 200–206
  nutritional profile, 201, 226
warfarin (Coumadin), 18,
  182–83

weight control
    avocado and, 137
    broccoli and, 160
    coconut and, 65–66
    fruits and, 12, 17–18, 39
    green tea and, 165–66
    nuts and, 112–13, 131–32,
        205, 227–28
    wheat grass (*Triticum*
        aestivum), 71–77
When in Doubt, Eat Broccoli
    (Pearson), 158
Wilcox, Michael, 46
Willett, Walter C., 107
Wolfe, Robert R., 86

X

xeronine, 19
X Factor Holdings, 28–29

Z

zeaxanthin, 17, 101, 163
Zico Natural (coconut water), 25
zinc, 55, 220
The Zone Diet (Sears), 106